THE FASTING PHENOMENON

An Ancient Therapeutic Approach Toward Damaged Emotions and Traumatic Memories

By Dr. Curtis Ward DD MHC

Atria Book Publishing

A division of Atria House Publications

USA

Atria Book Publishing

A division of Atria House Publications

USA

ISBN: 978-0-615-26399-1

First published by Atria Book Publishing
October 2008.

Printed in the United States of America.

This book is printed on acid-free paper.

Dedication

To my precious wife, Rebecca, who stood by me during the midnight of my soul as I struggled with my own traumatic memories.

I will always be grateful to you for the many sacrifices you made while faithfully traveling abroad with me during the decades of our "glory years." These are precious memories I shall forever treasure.

Because of you I know angels still walk among men.

To my daughter, Makayla, and my son, Brandon, my rays of sunshine in a world full of darkness.

To you, the reader, may you find the peace of mind that you have so longed for and deserve.

CONTENTS

Preface

The sheer beauty of the theory presented within these pages flows so elegantly with what we know concerning the structure of nature, of man, and the teaching of the ancients, that it seems almost an insult to call it a theory.

It is so simple, so natural, and once understood, so obvious, that one almost blushes in not having recognized such a powerful tool much sooner.

Science is just now beginning to rigorously research the benefits of fasting upon the body, the mind, and the spirit of man. The ancients, however, attempted to educate us in these areas long ago.

The recent groundbreaking studies, which have produced stunning results in the laboratory, have been mostly limited to the effects of fasting on the physical organism.

However, the surprising discovery of the fasting method and its effects on the psyche has now emerged offering a revolutionary approach toward emotional problems.

You are about to read the printed results of that discovery.

In this book we will explore the effects of fasting on trauma and painful memories. We will discover how fasting can discharge the pent up emotions hidden in a memory of the past that may be unconsciously affecting your life today.

Chapter One will present a synopsis of this work and the chapters following will explore the history of those who tried and failed to find a cure for traumatic memories. This will be followed by an exploration of the nature of trauma, what we are searching for, and the ancient method that is still available to us today. The fasting method will then be presented in a simple user friendly version followed by a more in depth and detailed version (before personally attempting the fasting method please read disclaimer on page 100). Finally we shall hear the stories of those in whom the fasting method effected almost miraculous results.

Man has created both an environmental and a psychological imbalance of nature through his abusive misunderstanding of it. There is so much that man does not know about the wisdom that underlies all of nature and so much he thinks he knows.

Albert Einstein once said,

"The human mind is not capable of grasping the Universe. We are like a little child entering a huge library. The walls are covered to the ceilings with books in many different tongues. The child knows that someone must have written these books.

It does not know who or how.

It does not understand the languages in which they are written. But the child notes a definite plan in the arrangement of the books

—a mysterious order which it does not comprehend—

but only dimly suspects."

Chapter One

Damaged Emotions

Have you ever suffered from depression lasting more than three days?

Have you ever had anxiety that prevented you from functioning as you wished you could?

Has something in your past haunted you and prevented you from achieving the happiness and success in life that you know you are capable of achieving?

If you answered *"yes"* to any of the above questions, you may be suffering from emotional and mental trauma in one or more of its varied forms.

Today, more than at any other time in history, people are plagued with stress, depression, and feelings of hopelessness. The counselor's office is full and in order to book a psychiatrist one must schedule an appointment months in advance. The mental health profession has become so overwhelmed that it is now very common to hear of the

1

family doctor prescribing medications which, in most cases, were formerly left in the hands of the psychiatric office.

Just a few decades ago we were told we didn't need drugs — we just needed to understand our childhood. Today we are told we don't need to understand our childhood — we just need drugs. One of the most prescribed drugs in the world today is Prozac.

Prozac, and its chemical cousins, are not only the most prescribed drugs in the world, but the most prescribed drugs in all of medical history. Prozac is bringing home the bacon for the pharmaceutical industry at the merry tune of over 3 billion dollars a year. More than 28 million people in the United States, almost one in ten Americans, take antidepressants.

In the United States alone over 2.7 million prescriptions for antidepressants are written annually to children from ages 1 to 11. There are over 8.1 million prescriptions for antidepressants annually written for teens from ages 12 to 17. [1]

Although an alarming number of people are in treatment for depression, it is estimated that depression will very soon be the world's second-most-disabling disease (after heart disease) no later than the year 2020. [2]

Amazingly, one out of every six Americans uses tranquilizers regularly. Over 250 million prescriptions are written a year for the highly addicting, cognitive impairing benzodiazepines (tranquilizers) such as Xanex and Valium. [3]

Electroconvulsive therapy treatments (shock treatments) are routinely administered to a conservative estimate of 100,000 Americans annually.[4] An ad for the most widely used shock machine tells doctors they need only set a dial to a patient's age and press a button. [5]

Marianne Ueberschar, of Toronto, checked herself into the city's Centre for Addiction and Mental Health suffering from severe depression.

Like many older women entering psychiatric wards in Canada, Ueberschar, now 69, was offered electroconvulsive shock therapy, or ECT. She refused, and fought a legal battle with the institution to prevent it from administering the treatment.

"I said I don't want my brains fried, thank you very much," says Ueberschar, who was discharged five months later without having been hooked up to electrodes to induce a generalized seizure. [6]

More than 500 lobotomies are performed yearly in just the United States. [7] A patient goes to the mental institution haunted by a past of sexual and physical abuse and is put to sleep while a piece of her/his brain is sliced up by the surgeon.

Alcohol abuse and drug addiction has risen to an all time high. A greater percentage of alcoholics and drug abusers claim their addiction began as a way of escaping some horrible trauma . . . some abuse done to them . . . something they themselves did and have never forgiven themselves for . . . some memory that unrelentingly torments them like a demon from Hades.

Our young men graduate from high school with precious dreams of making something great out of their lives. Many enlist in the armed forces and bravely do their best to serve their country. Many come home very different than they were when they left. Many will bring home a reminder of war called "post traumatic stress disorder" (formerly referred to as shell shock). They will be forced to endure a lifetime of haunting nightmares, flashbacks, feelings of depression, anxiety, feeling numb, feeling detached from others, being easily startled, and being haunted with remorse and fear.

Untold millions just this year alone will self medicate their experience of being raped, molested, and physically or emotionally abused with prescriptions borrowed from friends, with prescriptions purchased through some dubious company over the Internet, or with an over-the-counter drug such as Nyquil.

Pills, shock treatments, lobotomies, booze . . . it makes no difference if you pop it, shock it, snip it, or sip it. The problem usually remains.

Is it possible that an ancient remedy from the distant past could hold the answer for millions of sufferers?

Could the answer lie within the pages of a manuscript, written many millennia ago by sages and prophets, that we today refer to as the "Holy Bible?" Could the very answer lie in plain sight within the chapel room of the very hospital in which the surgeon, in another room, is hacking a piece of a sufferer's brain or shocking her/him into a convulsive seizure?

I propose that the most powerfully effective healing for

trauma, depression, debilitating memories, and a host of many other conditions which are plaguing millions around the world is the ancient tried and proven art of fasting.

What?

That's right . . . fasting.

"Fasting?" you may ask. *"Isn't fasting abstinence from food? Isn't that what all these religious and health food fanatics do?"*

It is true fasting has, in the past, been mostly relegated to religious and health conscious circles. But today, more than ever, it is coming under the scrutiny of modern science. What was once observed in the hidden mountain hideaway by the observant ascetic is now being observed in the modern laboratory.

Studies have shown the benefits of fasting in slowing the aging process, rejuvenation, and producing many other almost miraculous benefits. It may also be the most powerful healing tool for damaged emotions that has ever existed. As a matter of fact, in some cases, it may be the only cure.

I am neither advocating nor denouncing the above-mentioned therapies utilized by the medical profession. There are those who will never search for a natural therapy and medication or shock treatments may be the only thing standing between them and suicide.

BUT there IS a better way . . . a natural way . . . a permanent cure.

This powerful tool became very apparent to me after decades of observing other therapies fail in removing the emotional conflicts so stubbornly embedded within the minds of numerous sufferers. I observed sufferers in which no amount of therapy seemed to ameliorate their pain. In contrast I witnessed some of these, who utilized the art of fasting and prayer, make remarkable recoveries such as has never been witnessed by medical science.

My suspicions were that fasting was a healing science for traumatic memories and that the Creator had designed man in such a way as to respond positively to it. It was this conviction that compelled me to research this subject more in depth.

FASTING EFFECTS ON MENTAL ILLNESS

Fasting has been known for some time to have some very profound effects on mental illness.

Previously fasting has been studied for its normalizing and stabilizing effect on nervous and mental functions. Dr. Alan Cott went to Russia to study under Professor Yuri Nikolayev who was experiencing a very high success rate for treatment of chronic refractory schizophrenia. In 1972, Professor Nicolayev, director of the fasting unit of the Moscow Psychiatric Institute, reported on the use of scientifically therapeutic fasting to successfully treat more than 7000 patients, all suffering from neuropsychiatric disorders such as schizophrenia and various other nervous disorders. Professor Nicolayev said, *"The hunger treatment* [the Russian psychiatric term for "fasting"] *gives the entire nervous system and the brain a rest. The body is also cleansed of poisons, and the tissues and the various glands are renovated. Resting of the brain forms the basis for the treatment of various neuropsychiatric disorders. Treatment through fasting is an internal operation, without a scalpel."* [8]

Allan Cott, M.D., wrote in "Fasting: The Ultimate Diet", *"Seventy percent of those treated by fasting improved so remarkably that they were able to resume an active life."* (pp 34-35). Dr. Cott further writes: *"An epochal breakthrough in the treatment of schizophrenia came when Doctor Nikolayev discovered that his patients responded to fasting treatment after all other forms of therapy had failed."* (p 34) [9]

While amazed with this information, I still had to ask myself, *"Could fasting also, in some unexplained way, affect emotions damaged by former trauma?"*

TRAUMATIC MEMORIES RESISTANT TO THERAPY

Post traumatic stress disorder and other types of trauma have proven to be particularly resistant to both therapy and medication. Various methods have been devised in an attempt to reach the memory of trauma embedded within the circuits of the human brain.

Eye movement desensitization and reprocessing (EMDR) is a therapeutic technique discovered by therapist Dr. Francine Shapiro in which the patient moves her/his eyes back and forth rapidly, while concentrating on the traumatic and disruptive memory. The therapist waves an object in front of the patient. The patient is supposed to follow the object with her/his eyes to simulate the movement of REM (Rapid Eye Movement).[10] The therapist then gives commands to the client to release the traumas and emotions that are surfacing, and these are al-

7

legedly released via the eyes through rapid blinking. Results to date have been moderate.

Hypnotism has been used as a therapeutic tool by putting the client in a trance and commanding her/him to remember the tormenting event as it occurred. Results with this treatment have been even less successful.

Psychoanalysis has been used in a similar method in which the analysand (the patient) closes her/his eyes, remembers the troublesome event, and allegedly releases the emotional charge by rehearsing the memory to the analyst. Most mental health professionals today believe this technique to be ineffective.

As mentioned above, electric shock treatment and lobotomy have been utilized in attempt to temporarily erase the tormenting memories many people suffer with.

Researchers are searching frantically for a drug that will access the forbidden area in the human brain where these memories hide and delete the emotive energy.

THE NEGLECTED SOLUTION

In the face of such a great dilemma an innovative discovery has now been unveiled that releases the horrible hold these ingrained memories have upon its victims.

It is such a natural and simple method, that the concept evaded me for years. My suspicions about the beneficial effects of fasting on traumatic memories, which initially spurred my research into this intriguing subject,
resulted in a theoretical paradigm which has repeatedly demonstrated dramatically successful results.

Recent laboratory research studies on fasting have inadvertently validated the core elements of this theoretical paradigm.

At last there is a workable solution for millions of sufferers.

The primary theory of this discovery teaches that during a crisis the mind enters the state of trauma in which a highly charged memory is imprinted on the sensitized brain. This imprinted memory becomes a survival mechanism that prepares the individual to fight or flee should a similar situation arise. However, this mechanism does not work efficiently within modern technological societies.

To release the emotional charge, one must revisit the trauma while in a hypersensitive state similar to trauma. During this experience the emotion of the event is discharged, and the area that the trauma previously occupied is reprogrammed with a healthy view of the event.

This hypersensitive state similar to trauma is the fasting experience.

During fasting the body is traumatized by severe food abstinence and in an effort to survive it switches the brain and senses into a hypersensitive mode. When in this state of trauma the individual is instructed to intentionally revisit the memory, and the emotion of the event is discharged and changed through the simple reprogramming method which we will outline later in another chapter.

There is no need for hypnotism, analysis, or rapid eye movement. Neither medication nor electroshock treatments are involved. Only the natural scientific art of fasting is utilized in retrieving, discharging, and reprogramming the traumatic memories.

It is virtually IMPOSSIBLE for ANYONE, including the reader, to live in today's world without having experienced some measure of damaged emotions or hurt from the past

Untold multitudes are suffering from various emotional pains and millions of others are being treated unsuccessfully with various therapeutic measures, some very damaging and intrusive, to no avail. As previously mentioned, millions more are self medicating their hurt with alcohol, crack, marijuana, and other drugs. The alarming increase of the world percentage of psychiatric patients indicates the need for a more thorough therapeutic tool. The ancient art of fasting may just be what the doctor didn't but should have ordered.

In the next two chapters we will examine the historical medical search for such cures. Then we will examine the biology of trauma and damaged emotions, and finally we will explore how fasting can ameliorate these impediments with details of how the method works. The information may just change your life.

Chapter Two

The Search for a Cure:

Looking Inside the Brain

One weekend Robert Henderson had a large hole drilled through his skull.

He had read that this procedure, known as trepanation, could rid him of tormenting memories from the past. He was haunted by events that he experienced as a child and often found himself in the depth of depression. After several months of discussing the procedure with friends, watching surgical videos and documentaries, going to libraries and doing personal research, as well as attending an actual viewing of a trepanation, he decided he would go ahead and have the procedure performed and began searching for ways to achieve his goal.

"I have suffered with extreme depression my whole life," Robert said, *"Depression would overshadow me like a dark cloud. I'd be feeling normal and all of a sudden be so depressed I wanted to die."*

"I tried everything" Robert said, *"Therapy, hypnotism, antidepressants . . . you name it! Nothing helped."*

"It was perpetual torment," Robert added, *"My counselor said it was because of my past, things I experienced in my childhood. My family was dysfunctional. My dad came home one night in a drunken rage and said he was going to kill Mom. I believed him. He started beating her. I saw blood. She fell on the floor and I thought for sure she was dead. I ran upstairs and hid in the closet. I shook until I finally fell asleep from exhaustion. I was awakened the next morning by Dad pulling me out of the closet. He calmed me down telling me he loved me. I went down-stairs and there was Mom and my brothers and sisters, all sitting at the breakfast table smiling like everything was normal. I never got over that experience. Death always seemed right around the corner."*

"After years of torment I became desperate for relief," Robert said.

Trepanation is a surgical procedure in which a permanent hole is drilled though the skull. First a flap of skin is cut and folded back. Then a piece of the skull is removed, leaving the durra mater of the brain exposed. The flap of skin is then replaced back and stitched over the top of the wound. After healing, there remains a "soft spot" similar to that which a baby is born with. However, in a baby the soft spot is soon covered with a new growth of bone. In an adult new bone does not grow over it and the individual is left with a permanent soft spot. It is believed that this hole allows the brain to "breath" and pulsate normally and ultimately rid the patient of depression and tormenting memories. Primitive tribes in third world countries   perform ceremonial trepanations believing that the surgery produces a place in the skull for the demon, responsible for the patient's woes, to escape. Herbert Hughes, the man originally responsible for coming up with the modernized theory of trepanation, taught that a hole in the head allowed the brain to pulsate with the rest of the bodies rhythm. Unbelievably many people accepted his theory. We will take a closer look at "Doctor" Hughes' credentials later.

One woman, driven by depression and unable to find a doctor in America to do the surgery, made a trip to Mexico where it is legal for a physician to perform the operation. After her surgery, she claimed to have some relief from depression. This is most probably a simple placebo effect such as some patients experience when given a "sugar pill." Believing they have taken medicine they begin to improve. In other words the beneficial results were "all in her head."

Robert is only one of many that have sought this bizarre answer to ridding themselves of the dark cloud of despair and, like the woman mentioned above, Robert could not find a doctor to perform the trepanation, so he began to search for someone on the Internet. He located the name of a man that had performed the procedure on himself. Communicating first by email and then by telephone, he soon became well acquainted with this man (whom we will refer to as Duane) and, after a few months after his initial contact with him, asked him to assist in performing the trepanation. Duane, a high school drop out, came to Robert's home and they made a list of things needed to do the surgery.

They purchased a drill and autoclaved bits from the hardware store and sterile gauze, antiseptic wipes, and other paraphernalia from the home medical supply store. Together with some of Robert's friends they prepared for the surgery to be done in Robert's upstairs bedroom. They sterilized the drill and bits with alcohol and set them on a tray beside of them. A flashlight washed in alcohol, the sterile wipes, sodium chloride to wash the wound, and other needed instruments were placed beside the drill and bits. Plastic sheets were laid down on the floor and a large sheet placed on the nearest wall where the procedure was to take place. They were ready to go.

After shaving Roberts head, disinfecting the area, and removing the skin, they fired up the drill. Duane placed his weight against the drill as the screaming bit chewed through Robert's skull. The grisly sound, combined with a mist of blood, caused Robert's girlfriend to faint. The procedure had to be delayed until she was brought to consciousness. After she had calmed down, they disinfected the area again, and proceeded with surgery.

I will spare you the rest of the lurid details. Suffice it say it was not a pretty scene to behold.

It took some time for the wound in Roberts head to heal. At first he was pleased with the results believing his depression had been alleviated. But he was to soon be disappointed when the dark cloud of depression descended again, smothering any hope of being freed from his perpetual curse.

As mentioned earlier, Dr. Bart Hughes (b. 1934) was the man responsible for devising and promoting the modern theory of trepanation. Dr. Hughes was a medical school graduate who had never practiced medicine except for self-surgery, and was commonly referred to as "Doctor" although he never completed his medical degree. He said that he wanted to be a psychiatrist but had failed his medical exam and therefore never went into practice. Dr. Hughes taught that trepanation increases "brain blood volume" and thereby enhances cerebral metabolism in a manner that is similar to cerebral vasodilators such as the herb ginkgo biloba. He relates that his first insight came when he was taught that he could obtain higher consciousness and a "natural high" by standing on his head. He came to the conclusion that by permanently relieving pressure, he could increase blood flow to the brain thus streamlining the human brain to work more efficiently. [11]

Thus, was born the modern theory of trepanation.

It would have been much more beneficial to have just taken ginkgo biloba and stood on his head.

There is no shortage of modern practitioners of trepanation claiming its medical benefits as a treatment for depression and other psychological ailments. On April 10, 2001, it was reported that two Cedar City Utah men pleaded guilty to practicing medicine without a license after it was discovered they had drilled holes into a woman's skull in an attempt to treat her symptoms of depression and chronic fatigue syndrome. Peter Halvorson, 54, and William Lyons, 56, were placed on three years' probation, fined $500 and ordered to undergo psychiatric evaluation. The woman, however, claimed to have received some relief from her symptoms. [12]

The International Trepanation Advocacy Group is an organization that advocates the questionable procedure originally promoted by Dr. Hughes teaching. Many are listening to their message as a last resort. [13]

The surgery has no scientific grounds and all evidence suggests it has no beneficial effects on health. It is a high risk procedure for permanent brain damage, infection, sepsis, and certain death.

Many today, desperate for relief, continue to follow such absurd and extreme pseudo-sciences such as trepanation. A man in England was so devastated by emotional trauma that he decided on trepanation as his only answer. He was found dead with the drill still in his hands.

The modern popularity of this unproven and very dangerous technique is ample evidence that available therapies and medications are not sufficiently alleviating the emotional pain nor meeting the needs of the people.

There IS a much less painful, much more natural, and a more scientifically grounded answer.

It involves absolutely no surgery, cutting, nor scarring. In fact the nonsurgical, natural art of fasting has been known to REDUCE scar tissue that has been present in the human body for decades. [14] Such a simple answer has been available since the beginning of time. Yet people have been consistently drawn to such bizarre and radical surgeries as mentioned above.

While trepanation may seem unbelievably bizarre, we will next explore a procedure that is just as bizarre, if not more so. It is a surgery that not only makes a hole in the head but actually severs the tissue in the brain. It is legal, it is done by medical doctors, and in times past has been forced upon patients.

It is known as lobotomy.

LOBOTOMY

Medical doctors in search of a permanent cure for debilitating depression and damaged emotions, discovered that slicing portions of brain matter seemed to calm these previously agitated individuals.

The first attempts at human psychosurgery in the twentieth century occurred in 1935, when neurosurgeons Egas Moniz and Almeida Lima at the University of Lisbon, began performing a series of prefrontal lobotomies — a procedure in which the connection between the prefrontal cortex and the rest of the brain is severed. [15] Originally the procedure involved drilling holes in the patient's head and destroying tissue in the frontal lobes by injecting alcohol. Now doesn't that sound like a pleasant procedure? He later improved the technique using a leucotome, an instrument that cut brain tissue with a retractable wire loop.

The neurosurgeons claimed fair results, most notably in the treatment of depression, although about 6 per cent of patients did not survive the operation. That didn't sound like such a bad percentage UNLESS you were part of that 6 per cent! There were often adverse changes in the patient's personality and social interactions. Despite the obvious risks, the procedure took hold with a faddish zeal as it was promoted as the answer to curing mental conditions.

This barbaric science left multitudes of disabled people and deaths in its path.

17

In 1949 Egas Moniz, highly praised for his work in lobotomy, received the coveted Nobel Prize.

Is something wrong with this picture?

ICE PICK LOBOTOMY

Walter Freeman popularized psychosurgery when he invented the "ice pick lobotomy." This surgery consisted of literally using an ice pick and a rubber mallet instead of standard surgical equipment to perform a transorbital lobotomy. [16]

In the early 1940s, he took an ice pick from his own kitchen and began to test the new surgical technique on cadavers. The very next year he began practicing on living patients. The patient was either anesthetized or rendered unconscious by electroshock treatment before the highly invasive surgery began. The technique involved lifting the upper eyelid and placing a leucotome, which was basically an ice pick, under the eyelid and against the top of the eye socket. Dr. Freeman would then hammer the ice pick into the patient's skull with a mallet just above the tear duct. After penetrating the skull, he began wiggling and twisting it into the brain. The leucotome was then moved from side to side, to sever the nerve fibers connecting the frontal lobes to the thalamus. Sometimes the bottom of the ice pick was pulled upward, sending the tip farther back into the brain and producing a deep frontal cut. The instrument was then withdrawn, and the procedure was repeated on the other side.

With the zeal of an evangelist Dr. Freeman, from 1936 through the 1950s, traveled the United States in his personal van, which he referred to as his "lobotomobile," demonstrating his newfound butchering technique everywhere he went. [17] Reportedly he performed procedures in various medical settings as well as in hotel rooms. [18]

Dr. Freeman's evangelical fervor quickly popularized the lobotomy as a general cure for all types of perceived impediments such as misbehavior in young children. If your kid acted up you simply bored a hole in his head, chopped some brain tissue, and the problem was solved. Obviously it was more difficult to persuade a child to go to the local lobotomist's office than it was to go to the local dentist. However, drilling a hole in your child's brain was more in vogue than drilling a hole in his tooth.

Reportedly Dr. Freeman's most notable failure was the prefrontal lobotomy he performed on Rosemary Kennedy, sister of the former President of the United States, which transformed her into an inert vegetable unable to speak more than a few words.

"What? Rosemary Kennedy?" you may ask, *"I had always heard she was born retarded!"*

That is what most of us have been led to believe. This is what the media projected, what the Medical Association preferred for us to believe, and what we have been fed wholesale for decades.

However, Rosemary's life has a different story to tell.

Rosemary was described as a shy child, but thoughts she logged in her diaries in the late 1930s and published in the 1980s, reveals a happy, sophisticated, curious, young woman whose life was filled with outings to the opera, tea dances, dress fittings, and various other social interests. She wrote the most lovely and endearing letters. Her writing was intelligent, insightful, sensitive, and at times very touching. She was far from being *"retarded"* as the public has been led to believe. [19]

Although easygoing as a child, she became increasingly assertive in her personality as she entered puberty. Observers maintain this behavior was a reaction to the challenge of keeping up with her siblings as well as the trauma of hormonal changes and mood swings commonly seen in many teenagers. The family had trouble dealing with the stormy natured girl which had begun to sneak out at night from the convent where she was being educated. Evidently they thought it was unnatural for a growing young girl to dislike being confined to a convent. When Rosemary turned 23, her father was told by her doctors that a lobotomy would help ease her *"mood swings that the family found difficult to handle at home."* Obviously they trusted the venerable position of the medical doctors in the same way that we trust the chemical pushing medical profession today.

Dr. James Watts, who with Dr. Freeman performed the procedure, wrote: *"We went through the top of the head, I think she was awake. She had a mild tranquilizer. I made a surgical incision in the brain through the skull. It was near the front. It was on both sides. We just made a small incision, no more than an inch."* The instrument Dr. Watts used looked like a butter knife. He swung it up and down to cut brain tissue. *"We put an instrument inside,"* he said. As Dr. Watts cut, Dr. Freeman put questions to Rosemary. For example, he asked her to recite the Lord's Prayer or sing *"God Bless America"* or count backwards . . . *"We made an estimate on how far to cut*

20

based on how she responded." When she began to become incoherent, they stopped. —James W. Watts [20]

When she became incoherent . . . they stopped . . .

When she became virtually brain dead . . .
they stopped . . .

When they flubbed up . . . they stopped . . . they stopped with Rosemary but they went on their merry way to barbarically butcher others.

Instead of making Rosemary a more manageable young woman, the lobotomy reduced Rosemary to an infantile mentality that left her incontinent, staring blankly at walls for hours, and mentally incapacitated for the rest of her life. She was confined to wearing diapers like a baby. Her verbal skills were reduced to an unintelligible babble. Mrs. Rose Kennedy, her mother, remarked that although the lobotomy stopped her daughter's stormy behavior, it left her completely incapacitated. *"Rose was devastated; she considered it the first of the Kennedy tragedies."* [21]

TRAUMA —NOT RETARDATION

John White, Kathleen Kennedy's former boyfriend, claimed Kathleen, the former Presidents sister, shared with him the very private family secret that Rosemary had suffered with *"mood changes,"* which was most disturbing to her father. She added that *"the family considered Rosemary a disgrace and failure',"* [22]

Rumors began to circulate that Rosemary had already been retarded before the surgery. As previously men-

21

tioned, this rumor was widely accepted and even today is still believed by the majority of the American public. Ronald Kessler, author of "The Sins of the Father," writes that Dr. Watts *"told the author that, in his opinion, Rosemary had suffered not from mental retardation, but from a form of depression . . . 'It may have been agitated depression . . . '"* [23]

The former director of the National Institute of Mental Health, Dr. Bertram S. Brown, said, *"If she did division and multiplication* [which she did], *she was over an IQ of 75. She was not mentally retarded. It could be she had an IQ of 90 in a family where everyone was 130, so it looked like retardation, but she did not fall into an IQ 75 and below, which is the definition of mental retardation . . . There is no way I can picture her at less than a 90 IQ, but in that family, 90 would be considered retarded."*

At the age of nine, she did problems like 428 x 32 = 13696, 3924 / 6 = 654. At age 16 she wrote to her father, *"I would do anything to make you so happy. I hate to disappoint you in any way."*

It was further Dr. Brown's opinion that the family's treatment of Rosemary is what led to her stormy emotional struggles. Kessler quotes Dr. Brown as saying, *"I think it's likely she was somewhat slower than the others. Then she was treated as if she was retarded. Then it becomes reactive depression, including rages and loss of control . . . that is mental illness . . . The reason she got depressed was that she reacted to being treated as a lesser member of the family."* While the children tried to include her in their social activities, *"given the highly competitive environment of the Kennedy family, they could not help but to communicate to her that she was not up to their standards."*

In light of these facts, it seems Rosemary was suffering from social TRAUMA. She was not good enough to be accepted by the rest of the family. There was great inner turmoil and pain. Embedded within her mind were various incidences in which she experienced being rejected and humiliated. It has been said that Joe's banishment of Rosemary to live with his aide was perceived by Rosemary as the pinnacle of utter rejection.

"The stigma of mental illness in those days," said Dr. Brown, *"was like tuberculosis or cancer or worse."* Dr. Brown called the suppression of the truth in this tragic story **"the biggest mental health cover-up in history."** Since the "public story" is still that Rosemary was retarded, the *"lack of support for mental illness is part of a total lifelong family denial of what was really so . . . Some of us knew the secret and kept it secret . . ."* [24]

After her lobotomy, the young girl that once poured graceful words into enduring letters and whose heart was filled with dreams — aspirations that every young person should have the chance to fulfill — was sent to live at St. Coletta's School in Wisconsin, where she remained, staring at walls and blubbering incoherently for the rest of her life. She quietly passed away on January, 7, 2005 at the age of 86.

Dr. Watts, who held the ice pick that severed the brain of the once young and very beautiful Rosemary, was highly respected and later became the 91st president of the Medical Society of the District of Columbia.

TAKE THREE ASPIRINS AND CALL ME
IN THE MORNING

You CANNOT cut out trauma and psychological pain from a section of the brain.

Facts indicate Rosemary suffered from trauma and not retardation. If this is indeed true, then we have been lied to about the tragic case of Rosemary Kennedy.

If we were lied to about Rosemary, what else has the medical world and the media lied to us about? We are expected to unquestioningly follow our doctor's orders, but can these orders always be trusted? Do they really have "the answer?" When they discover they are wrong will they stop and admit it?

THE LOBOTOMOBILE ROLLS ON

Dr. Watt and Dr. Freeman launched a scientific method that quickly caught fire. Lobotomists sprang up all over the world.

Between 40,000 and 50,000 patients were lobotomized in a very short period of time. A follow-up study of English lobotomies performed between 1942 and 1954 claimed 41% of patients had *"recovered"* or were *"greatly improved,"* 28% were *"minimally improved,"* and 25% showed *"no change,"* 4% had died, while 2% were made worse. [25] Of course these figures depend on what you define as *"greatly improved"* which may mean that a once very active young person was now more or less a vegetable. This was indeed a great improvement for parents who didn't want to parent or teachers who didn't want to teach. It was very similar to the present "chemical lo-

24

botomization" our children are being subjected to because of a scholastic system that has neither the patience to deal with its students nor the legal authority to reprimand them.

GIVE THE MEDICAL PROFESSION A PIECE OF YOUR MIND!

Lobotomies are STILL being performed TODAY— right now — in the enlightened twenty first century!

Modern day lobotomies are performed as a treatment for sufferers of resistant obsessive compulsive disorder, anorexia, and other treatment resistant mental conditions. The efficacy of the procedure, however, is not high: a study of cingulotomy (which involves a 2–3 cm lesion in the cingulum near the corpus callosum) found improvement in a mere 5 out of 18 patients. [26]

NINETEEN NINETY SEVEN

Guidelines for present day lobotomies according to Kaplan and Sadock (1997):

"A reasonable guideline is that the disorder should have been present for 5 years . . . "

"Chronic intractable major depressive disorder and obsessive-compulsive disorder are two disorder's reportedly most responsive to psychosurgery."

"The major indication for psychosurgery (lobotomy) is the presence of a debilitating, chronic mental disorder that has not responded to any other treatment." [27]

OK, OK . . . lobotomy does not work for everyone. But if the area in the brain where these little demons from the past are stored can't be CUT out . . . then why can't they just be SHOCKED out?

ELECTROCONVULSIVE SHOCK TREATMENTS

One woman, raised by her abuser in a dysfunctional home, was so traumatized by her past that chronic depression had become a part of her everyday life. She didn't know what life without depression was. It was a part of her.

She checked herself into a mental institution in hope that she could find relief from her symptoms. The doctors prescribed electric shock treatments.

After leaving the hospital she returned home with virtually no depression.

She also returned with no memory as to whom her husband and children were.

She lost her job because she had no idea how to perform her previous duties. Decades of work experience had been erased. To compound matters, within two years after the final electroshock treatment, the chronic depression resurfaced.

Her job didn't. Neither did her husband who had filed for divorce and had moved on with his life.

WAYNE

Wayne Lax doesn't remember anything about his wedding day. There is no recall of his various suicide attempts. He doesn't remember much about his son. As a matter of fact there is not much of anything he remembers about his past.

Wayne's memory was damaged over a 25-year period in which he was admitted to the hospital 108 times, prescribed to take up to 17 pills a day, and was given 80 electroconvulsive shocks.

"I had more pills pumped into me than Elvis Presley."

He says his lower back was damaged when he wasn't given enough muscle relaxant before one of his shock treatments. At least 70 percent of his long-term memory was erased by the treatments which induce convulsive seizures in patients it is administered to.

During the entire time Wayne was suffering from untreated alcoholism.

"I was impaired on drugs, and they used to send me out to work," Wayne recalls.

His life took a dramatic turnaround in 1992 when he was involved in a car accident and lost his drivers license. With no way to support himself and realizing he was placing other people's lives in jeopardy, he was forced to reevaluate his own life. Wayne made the choice to give up the prescription drugs and electric shock treatments that had controlled his life for over 25 years.

"When I left the pills alone, the urge to drink left," he says.

He was left with a burning determination to help others who were going through the treatments administered by the same medical system he had managed to survive.

He has now dedicated his life to speaking out against the methods of the psychiatric system, and especially about the dangers of electroconvulsive therapy.

"I just want to help other people, because I lived in [Hades] for 25 years, and it put 30 people around me through [hades].

I was told I'd never live on my own," he says, *"and there were about 10 or 11 overdoses and attempts at suicide, and they'd just pump me out and send me home with more medication."*

He maintains that he is not against all doctors or all psychiatrists, but explains that some of them have become dangerous because they have too much power.

Wayne said one doctor *"was like God to me, he was like a father."*

Wayne is also not against medication, but he thinks it makes no sense to prescribe certain medications to alcoholics.

"They're giving you another addiction."

He is adamantly against electroconvulsive therapy under all circumstances.

"It's a barbaric treatment, and I'd like to see electroconvulsive therapy banned," he says. *"If shock is the answer, why are people in the system for 40 years?"* [28]

28

Had it not been for addiction counseling, self help groups and a great support system, especially his family; he feels he would never have survived to tell his story today.

THERESA

Theresa, 64, was a clinical psychologist who had helped countless patients cope with mental health issues but had never experienced them herself.

When she turned 59, a major depression set in. Her own psychoanalyst dumped her saying, *"I can't help you any more, you're too far gone. You're no longer my patient."* Theresa's colleagues recognized the symptoms of clinical depression and recommended hospitalization. *"The doctors were very condescending. There was no psychotherapy at all. They didn't believe in that. They only wanted to treat me with drugs,"* Theresa says.

When her depression didn't respond significantly to the medications, her doctor then prescribed electroconvulsive therapy. *"I was scared out of my wits,"* she says. When she opposed the planned shock treatments, her doctor declared her incapable of making her own decisions. Theresa contacted a rights adviser and a lawyer. After her recovery, Theresa asked the doctor why he'd pushed for the shock therapy. He said, *"Because it's the simplest and most direct way of getting the person better and getting them out of the hospital and freeing the hospital bed. My goal is to empty the beds."* Theresa says that the stigma of mental illness cost her several friendships. Theresa now takes the herbal supplement St. John's Wort and attends a mood disorders group. [29]

EBERT

A man from Columbus Ohio is not certain how many of his memories are missing. George Ebert, 58, is able to recall that during a tour with his family he felt the need to cleanse himself. He began to hitchhike from Columbus to Texas with his son on a search for God.

He ended up being taken to the Ohio psychiatric hospital where Ebert had his first experience, not with God, but with electroconvulsive therapy (electroshock treatments). The 15 treatments with the device, he said, left him temporarily unable to perform even the simplest of tasks and that it left him permanently unable to remember patches of his life.

"Afterwards, I was given a container of milk and I could not figure out how to hold it, and given a spoon and I didn't know what it was for," said Ebert. [30]

GAUDRAIN

Jerry Gaudrain says he endured almost 25 years of progressive memory loss, hallucinations, episodes of confusion and depression and blames shock treatments he underwent as the major source of his problem.

Gaudrain, who discovered his brother's dead body in their Kenora home, fell into a deep depression. He began to drink frequently — not every day, but in binges that lasted several days. He became suicidal. He ended up at Kenora hospital where he was initially diagnosed as suffering from a mild reactive depression.

Doctors at Winnipeg General Hospital — now the Health

Sciences Centre—authorized shock treatment. According to Gaudrain that electric shock treatment set him on a course of treatment he believes kept him ill for 25 years.

"With the ECT and all the drugs, you walk around like a zombie," he commented. *"I'm the one-in-a-million that comes out of it."* [31]

THE SHOCKING TRUTH

More then 100,000 people receive ECT every year nationally, according to the American Hospital Association.

ECT is essentially an electrical shock administered to the brain. The shock induces cerebral seizures that disrupt normal electrical activity in the brain. The patient is first given an intravenous anesthetic. After the patient is asleep, a muscle relaxant is intravenously administered and the patient is then fitted with an oxygen mask which delivers pure oxygen. An electrical shock is then applied to the scalp which shocks the patient into a seizure with muscle contractions. Seizure activity shocks the brain, convulsively changing electrical patterns and inducing other unknown changes. It usually lasts about one minute. The patient is awake five to 20 minutes after the procedure. Exactly what changes take place in the brain or what damages may take place in the brain or the neural pathways are not known. The only thing known for certain is that in most patients it produces a calming effect — as calm as a potato or a carrot!

ECT, once derided as a primitive and disruptive treatment for mental illness, has recently returned with a popular vengeance to the psychiatric mainstream, resulting in a public outcry for the state to monitor its use

31

more closely than almost any other medical procedure. Since its inception the treatment's technology has advanced significantly, yet state lawmakers, doctors and patients are speaking out in vigorous debates that has dredged up from the grave the lingering stigma from ECT's early days.

One of the core issues is that of informed consent, what patients know about ECT's effects, and whether they can be compelled to undergo it.

The battle is far from being over.

In one highly publicized case in 1999 on Long Island, Paul Henri Thomas challenged Pilgrim Psychiatric Center's right to administer electroshock treatments against his will. Pilgrim Psychiatric Center had to go to court to proceed with the treatment. The hospital won the case that March in favor of the hospital administering shock treatments against the patients will. [32]

We are often assured that ECT has advanced beyond the older, crude technology once used — but can we believe these reports?

While the individuals above (except for Ebert) were all given ECT by modern state of the art electroshock machines— there are some people who are not as fortunate. Unbelievably there are hospitals still using the archaic barbaric shock machines that was used during shock treatment's "dark days."

And there just may be more being used than you could ever guess.

SOME HOSPITALS STILL USE
DR. FRANKENSTIEN'S EQUIPMENT

Well, maybe not Dr. Frankenstein's . . . but it has recently been discovered some of the old equipment, which was part of yesterday's horror stories, are STILL being used today.

A recent study by the New York State Psychiatric Institute based at Columbia University revealed that some patients were still being treated with the archaic, outmoded ECT machines of yesteryear.

"Underscoring the absence of government oversight of ECT, state regulators said they do not know where these antiquated machines are, or even how many people receive ECT treatment . . . " writes Valerie Burgher of Newsday. [33]

Harold Sackeim, one of the authors of the study, refused to disclose the location of the hospitals still using the archaic machines of yesteryear, citing confidentiality of hospitals participating in the study. One is left to wonder what kind of antiquated machinery is used by hospitals not participating in this or other studies. One is further left to wonder if we should even give a hoot about their confidentiality when it comes to the personal health of the people.

Dr. John Oldham, of Columbia University's psychiatric research institute, said the sine wave shock machines may be less preferable than newer machines but they still deliver valuable treatment. *"The evolution of transitioning to improved medical and surgical equipment is a process,"* Oldham said. *"Hospitals can't immediately drop*

33

everything they've got. They have to do it in a planned, budgeted way."

Why of course! That makes reasonable sense. It would stress the budget even less to make it standard procedure that when a hospital's equipment breaks down, and they can't afford new equipment, to simply fly in a witch doctor from a third world country to perform trepanation by drilling holes in patients heads with a rhinoceros horn!

Gotta' watch that budget!

ONE FLEW OVER THE CUCKCOO'S NEST

"The American Psychiatric Association has been warning people not to use sine wave for 20 years or more, but they're still there," said Linda Andre, 41, of Manhattan, who underwent the treatment. Andre added that an independent agency should be formed to regulate ECT. She said psychiatrists *"didn't do anything"* to get rid of the sine wave machines before, and warned against having psychiatrists *"police"* themselves: *"You can't put these kinds of things in their hands."* [34]

I can almost hear McMurphy release an exasperated sigh. Some things never change.

SOMETIMES THERE SEEMS TO BE NO ALTERNATIVE

Sometimes patients are so completely overcome with depression, drowning in guilt, or languishing in the tormenting flames of the horrific memories of being molested, raped, or physically and mentally abused that it seems there may be no other alternative than shock therapy.

"The truth of the matter is that this [ECT] is now very routine," said Dr. Charles Kellner, professor of psychiatry and neurology at the Medical University of South Carolina. *"Some of them would die by suicide if people are denied access to this,"* he continues.

Is electroshock therapy indeed a necessary evil?

GOLF WAR TRAUMA

The following description of a woman who was treated for Post Traumatic Stress Syndrome (PTSD) with ECT appeared in The American Journal of Psychiatry:

"Ms. A was a 35-year-old married woman with a history of PTSD and depression. She reported feeling "on edge," with a sense of impending doom, since returning from active duty in the Persian Gulf war in 1991. Since then, she has had suicidal thoughts nearly every day. Although she has a family, she feels unable to achieve emotional closeness with others. During the gulf war, she was raped and witnessed numerous atrocities. She has reexperienced these events in the context of nightmares and daytime flashbacks, which are often triggered by certain odors such as diesel fuel and exhaust fumes.

In the past, several different pharmacotherapy regimens had been instituted without success . . . [then] she was placed on a regimen of sertraline (100 mg/day). According to Ms. A, this allowed her to "make it through the day," but it did nothing to alleviate her emotional numbness and hypervigilance. In the past, she had also been

35

treated with psychotherapy at a VA-sponsored PTSD clinic for women, without success.

Recently, Ms. A was admitted to our service because she felt her symptoms had escalated to the point that she was unable to continue living. She agreed to undergo ECT because her previous responses to pharmacotherapy and psychotherapy were inadequate. Ms. A underwent six unilateral ECT treatments, which were administered 3 times per week . . . After the third treatment, she reported feeling much better, with significant amelioration of her depression, emotional numbness, and recurrent intrusive thoughts . . . " (Helsey, Scott, PH.D, Tasmina Sheikh, MD, Kye Y. Kim, MD, and S.K. Park, MD, Buffalo, The American Journal of Psychiatry,1999) [35]

Ms. A was released on a regime of sertraline and discharged to go home where she could enjoy being with her family. We are not informed if there was a follow up on her case or how long her beneficial results may have lasted.

Although in the above case ECT was employed with at least some results, we are informed this is rare and that treating trauma with ECT commonly has extremely limited results and that the trauma usually returns after a period of time.

We are further told, *"PTSD is a common disorder with high comorbidity and a tendency toward chronicity, which RESPONDS SLOWLY TO TREATMENT and, in many patients, may not totally resolve EVEN WITH LONG-TERM TREATMENT."* (Sutherland SM, Davidon Jr., Department of Psychiatry, Duke University Medical Center, Durham, North Carolina) [36]

We further discover that *"both pharmacotherapy and psychotherapy often have LIMITED therapeutic outcomes in the treatment of PTSD."* [37]

One report informs us that, *"Drug studies show a modest but clinically meaningful effect on PTSD"* and that *"stronger effects were found for behavioral techniques involving direct therapeutic exposure"* but unfortunately *"severe complications have also been reported from the use of these techniques."* The report continues to say that studies of techniques including *"hypnosis suggest that these approaches may also hold promise."* [38]

So we have discovered that ECT has been used for post traumatic stress disorder. While in the case of Ms. A it was the only treatment that had any effect at all, the procedure hasn't demonstrated much success in other cases of trauma and when it has had some success it usually is not long lasting. We further discover that PTSD responds slowly to ANY type of treatment even if long-term. We also discovered that medication and talk therapy often have a LIMITED outcome. Finally we find that HYPNOTISM, of all things, may hold a promise in alleviating trauma. It seems we are coming back full circle to Mesmer and Puységur again!

Why would hypnotism even be remotely reconsidered?

Because researchers KNOW trauma is hidden somewhere in a dark realm of the inner mind. They just don't know how to reach it.

Sometimes in desperation, people are willing to do anything, including shocking their brain into seizures, to stop the inner torment

I reiterate: Is electroshock therapy indeed a necessary evil?

When all else fails, is this the only route to take—to shock the brain and wipe out the memory?

Is there perhaps another way to reach these areas of inaccessible pain that are so resistant to multiple therapeutic approaches?

When scientists finally climb to the top of the mountain of scientific achievement will they find the spiritually inspired ancients already there waiting to greet them?

Could the ancients have already discovered the secret to rejuvenation and healing of mind, body, and spirit?

Instead of looking for the answer in research papers and sterile laboratories, could the answer lie within an inspired manuscript too long neglected by the very scientists that are searching for the ancient wisdom it contains?

THE CHEMICAL LOBOTOMY:
PROZAC, VALIUM, AND SPEED . . . OH MY!!!

In May of 2005 representatives of mental health and consumer advocacy groups from throughout the USA held a peaceful protest and press conference in front of the headquarters of the Pharmaceutical Manufacturers and Researchers of America (PhRMA).

They said, *"The drug industry has taken over the mental*

health system. And we want it back."

Krista Erickson, board member of Mind Freedom International, says we should *"tell PhRMA to stop supporting forced psychiatric drugging! Tell PhRMA to be truthful about the clinical trials and side-effects of medications that their member companies are profiting from!"* [39]

Attorney Jim Gottstein, who has launched an investigation of the pharmaceutical industry, said, *"PhRMA represents the Big Lie of Big Pharma, which should be called to account for its despicable sacrifice of people on the altar of corporate profits."*

In addition to condemning the involuntary administration of psychotropic drugs to patients, he alleges that the pharmaceutical industry is misrepresenting the true nature of research findings on psychotropic drugs and covering up the evidence of harmful adverse effects they have and the hazards they create.

We do not need to repeat the stories of adverse effects from the futile use of medications that the above-mentioned ECT patients suffered with. While medication may have its proper place, its proper place is NOT in the hands of the pharmaceutical industry.

Must we remind people about the great cash inflow the industry benefited from with the release of the morning sickness miracle pill thalidomide? It was sold from 1956 to 1961 in the United States and almost 50 other countries. It was promoted, pushed, and prescribed to pregnant women as anti-emetic to combat morning sickness and as an aid to help them sleep. It had been tested before its release and the pharmaceutical company gave their full assurance that it was indeed a safe medication to take. They failed to mention that research had been a little rushed in order to get the drug out before Christmas, which was their prime time for selling new medications. Thousands of young mothers put their trust in the medical and pharmaceutical industry which resulted with catastrophic consequences for the children of these young women who had taken thalidomide during their pregnancies. From 1956 to 1962, this nightmare drug was responsible for more than 10,000 children born with severe deformities because their mothers had taken thalidomide during pregnancy. Some were born without arms. Some were born without legs. Women gave birth to children that were described as looking more like frogs, aliens, or amphibians than humans. Babies were born with flippers, like seals. There were so many deformities they are too numerous to list here. Recently the pharmaceutical drug from Hades has again reared its ugly head, with the appearance of its horrifying effects being passed on to the children of its former victims. This latest threat of possible litigation has the pharmaceutical company crying, *"No fair!"* It was reported in the British Sunday Mirror that six young men, who were born deformed because of thalidomide, have now fathered babies that have also been born with malformed limbs. Two of the babies have deformities almost identical to their fathers. Dr. William McBride, the Obstetrician that was the first to warn against thalidomide in 1961, says there are also second generation victims in Germany, Japan and Bolivia as well as Britain.

We trusted medical and pharmaceutical authorities with our children during the thalidomide years.

Should we trust them now during the Ritalin years?

In the United States alone, physicians are freely prescribing the mind-altering drug Ritalin to more than 2.2 million children each year.

Do we EVER learn?

Earlier we discussed the lobotimization of children who had alleged behavior problems. Today we have another bright answer for parents who don't want to parent or teachers who don't want to teach. We provide "chemical lobotomization" of our children with high doses of speed in order to vegetize normally bright, active children whom, as mentioned previously, teachers do not have the patience to deal with nor the legal authority to reprimand. Doctors today are prescribing these "behavior modifying" medications with just as much zeal as Dr. Freeman had in prescribing lobotomies.

Some of these children are simply active, curious children.

Some are traumatized.

A child lives in a dysfunctional family, is beaten, molested, or emotionally abused and she/he is given speed to correct the problem.

Adults are being medicated with just as an intense evangelical fervor as are the children. One medical doctor was discovered to have prescribed Prozac to EVERY SINGLE PERSON IN HIS COMMUNITY. He was later dubbed the "Prozac Doctor."

A woman is raped and is in the depths of depression. She is given a pill. Someone is beaten repeatedly by her husband. She is given a pill. A man returns home from the war with shell shock. He is given a pill. A woman remembers seeing her mother murdered by an intruder and still suffers with the memory. She is given a pill.

Do they have a pill for someone who is sick and tired of people whose only answer to a problem is to medicate it with a pill?

There are without a doubt some revolutionary discoveries in the area of chemical imbalances, neurotransmitters, and selective serotonin reuptake inhibitors. There are some legitimate, almost miraculous medications that have been discovered.

But do we need to indiscriminately prescribe and pass them out like Halloween candy to everyone that passes through our door?

Some medications are nothing more than band aides covering an emotional wound that needs healed. Can Xanex REALLY solve the core problem producing panic attacks? Can Valium really heal the pain of a man who was molested as a child by another man? Can a sleeping pill really dissolve the conflict that prevents a troubled mind from falling asleep?

Can Ativan or Valium really solve the inner confusion of a woman raped by someone she trusted?

There IS an answer.

It is natural.

It is free . . . and it works!

But the obvious has seemed to escape the majority.

We have discussed the search for a cure as we have observed individuals who have drilled holes in their own head, have allowed doctors to slice their brain with an ice pick, have had their brain electrified into convulsive seizures, and have consumed pain killing medications.

In the next chapter we shall continue observing the frantic search for a cure, however this time the search will not be that of how to alter the organic brain, but the search will take us deep within the mysterious, dark inner realms known as the subconscious mind.

Chapter three

The Search for a Cure
Looking Inside the Subconscious Mind

The ancients knew that there was "something" that seemed to "live" inside certain individuals and that this "something" drove them, ruled them, and caused them to produce some very strange behaviors. Various methods were devised to exorcize this "something." While the devil might indeed have been in the details, the fact of the matter is the devil had long gone and left his scars in the form of a psychological disorder and all the exorcism in the world couldn't exorcize something that needed HEALED.

In the New Testament it is recorded that they brought to Christ "all sick people that were taken with *diverse diseases* and *torments*, and those which were *possessed* with devils, and those which were *lunatick*, and those that had the *palsy*; and he healed them" (Matt. 4:24). One day while reading this verse, it suddenly dawned on me that there were five classes of people he healed:

1. *Diverse diseases* (many different kinds of physical illnesses),
2. *Torments* (those not possessed with, but tormented by demons),
3. *Possessed,* (possessed by demons),
4. *Lunaticks* (psychological problems and inner trauma's, NOT demon possession which had already been listed separately), and
5. *Palsy* (Neurological disorders).

I noticed that psychological problems and inner traumas were listed SEPARATELY from all the other illnesses — including possession. He did not exorcize "demons" from those with psychological struggles.

Most cultures around the world, however, have embraced exorcizing traumatic memories or have attempted to ameliorate the suffering by burning sacrifices to a sun or moon deity. They just knew that "something" was there. They just didn't know what or where.

There is a grand history of modern attempts to understand the anomalous, evasive world of inner conflicts.

It has long been suspicioned that there was a place in the psyche, somewhere in the mind itself, where past hurts were subconsciously hiding and tormenting its victim.

Several great minds have attempted to enter this mysterious inaccessible zone of the human mind. Earlier we briefly mentioned a few of them whom we will now revisit in more detail. They came close to closing in on the elusive creature prowling through the dark inner jungles of the subconscious mind.

One man, based on his understanding of Christian scriptures, ignited a fire that illuminated the path destined to become the mental science we know today as Psychology. His name was Juan Luís Vives.

JUAN LUÍS VIVES

Vives (1492-1540), as a small child, saw his father, grandmother, great-grandfather, and other members of his family, executed during the slaughter of the Jews during the Spanish Inquisition.

Vives' study of the life of Christ led him to accept Christianity and he later studied in Paris and was appointed professor of humanities at the University of Leuvain. He was a close friend of the great Christian theologian Erasmus who once said of him, *"We have with us Juan Luís Vives, a Valencian, only 26 years of age but already well versed in all the philosophical subjects, who has made such strides in belles-lettres, eloquence, oratory and writing that I hardly know of anyone to compare with him."* Erasmus insisted Vives write his elaborate commentary on Saint Augustine's "De Civitate Dei." Soon afterward he went to England where he was tutor to the Princess Mary. While living in England, Vives resided at Corpus Christi College, Oxford, where he became a doctor of law and taught philosophy. He spoke openly against the king's divorce from Catherine of Aragon, which he did not consider biblically doctrinal, and as a result he lost royal favor and was imprisoned for a time within his own home.

Vives is considered to be the first scholar to directly analyze the psyche. He performed extensive counseling sessions with people, and noted the relation between their exhibition of affect, and the particular words and issues they were discussing. While it is unknown if Freud was familiar with Vives' work, Gregory Zilboorg, historian of psychiatry, referred to Vives as *"the god-father of psycho-analysis,"* (A History of Medical Psychology, 1941).

Some also consider his work to be the beginning of psychology itself. He was a vigorous and adventurous thinker, opposing the authority of Aristotle and the orthodox ideas of his time. His inspiration veered him away from the Greek philosophies, which had dominated the Church for centuries, and he attempted to extract a fresh understanding of the human mind and the soul solely from the Holy Scriptures. He also emphasized reason over tradition. He is considered the forerunner of Francis Bacon by his application of psychological inquiry and by his pragmatic testing of hypotheses. Vives produced one of the very first works on modern psychology. Vives' treatise "De Anima et Vita" (1538; On the soul and life) is still widely recognized as a foundational text in the study of the inner life of the human being. In Vives' view, in order to know the soul, one must study its functions and operations, a study that is founded on a thorough knowledge of the physical, material life in its varied forms. The third book of "De Anima et Vita," an examination of the passions, was also a significant factor in gaining Vives the prominent place as a precursor of modern psychology, thanks to its employment of self-observation and introspection. His works were to later influence Johann Gassner.

JOHANN JOSEPH GASSNER

Gassner (1727-1779) studied at Prague and Innsbruck and became an ordained priest. A few years later his health began to fail him; without success he consulted various physicians; suddenly he conceived the theory that his infirmities might be due to the influence of an adverse spiritual entity which might be cured by utilizing spiritual methods. His experiment proved to be immensely successful. He applied this method also on others and soon thousands came to him to be healed. The fame of these cures spread far and wide; he was invited to other places; everywhere he went he had the same success.

He would command the evil spirit to depart from the afflicted, in the name of the Lord Jesus. To determine if the illness had a natural cause or not, he commanded the spirit to indicate by some sign that it was indeed present in the body. Other tests were conducted to rule out an exclusive physical cause of illness. Only after exhaustive tests, determining there was no physical cause of illness, he made use of "expulsive exorcism." Royals, physicians, and scholars from all over the world, and others, gathered around him to see the marvels they had heard of. Official investigations and records were made, and competent witnesses testified to the extraordinary results. The University of Ingolstadt appointed a commission, and so did the Imperial Government; both resulted with the approval of Gassner's procedure. However, his results were never able to be duplicated by others.

Some believe Gassner had discovered an inner part of the mind where indeed a dark entity had played havoc. Gassner's ideas and techniques paved the way for one of the most colorful personalities to ever stir the European continent. His name was Franz Mesmer.

FRANZ MESMER

Franz Anton Mesmer (1734-1815) studied medicine at the University of Vienna and later established himself as a physician in Vienna. In 1774, inspired by Gassner whom he later opposed, he began a treatment in which he employed something he called *"animal magnetism."* In 1775 he was invited to present his theories before the Munich Academy of Science. Some view this moment as the beginning of dynamic psychiatry.

Mesmer treated his patient by sitting in front of the individual with his knees touching the patient's knees, pressing the patient's thumbs in his hands, and looking fixedly into the patient's eyes. Mesmer made *"passes,"* moving his hands from patient's shoulders and down along their arms. Many patients felt peculiar sensations or had convulsions that were regarded as crises and supposed to bring about the cure.

An English physician who observed Mesmer said, *"The most sensible effects are produced on the approach of Mesmer, who is said to convey the fluid by certain motions of his hands or eyes, without touching the person. I have talked with several who have witnessed these effects, who have convulsions occasioned and removed by a movement of the hand . . . "*

Curing an insane person involved causing a fit of madness. One of the advantages of his method was the acceleration of such crises without danger.

49

It was from his method we derive the word "mesmerize" when referring to someone being hypnotized or influenced by charisma.

Evidently many who were affected by Mesmer's method were suffering from psychological disorders deep within that were responding to Mesmer's hypnotic therapy.

MARQUIS DE PUYSÉGUR

One of Mesmer's students, Marquis De Puységur (1751-1825), "mesmerized" one of his patients, Victor Race (a 23-year-old peasant employed by the Puységur family), with the result of Race entering an altered state of consciousness similar to sleepwalking. Race was very susceptible to becoming mesmerized into an altered state by Puységur, but displayed a strange form of sleeping trance that was not before seen in the early history of mesmerism. Puységur noted the similarity between this sleeping trance and natural sleepwalking (somnambulism). He named this state of consciousness as "artificial somnambulism."

This state was later renamed as the "hypnotic state" and the method in attaining it was called "hypnotism." The term hypnotism was coined in 1842 by James Braid.

Puységur rapidly became a highly successful hypnotherapist, to whom people came from all over France. Henri Ellenberger, the great historian of psychoanalysis and psychotherapy, wrote that Puységur was *"one of the great forgotten contributors to the history of the psychological sciences."* The details of the research of Puységur may be found in Ellenberger's master work, "The Discovery of the Unconscious," pp. 70-74.

Puységur's success in alleviating distress in his patients was his discovery of the existence of a "mind within the mind" that was largely unconscious. Today we know this as the subconscious mind. Puységur had stumbled unto one of the greatest discoveries of modern science. He had wandered into inner territory of the human psyche and, similar to Christopher Columbus, discovered the vast unexplored territory of the subconscious.

Unknowingly he tapped into the area where the brain had recorded emotional pain and traumatic events and, like a cook releasing steam from a cooker, was able to release some of the pent up energy associated with the stored memory. However, the inner conflict remained and the pressure slowly rebuilt, and the patient once again began suffering psychological symptoms.

Hypnotism was but a temporary fix and soon fell out of vogue. However, it was to be temporarily resurrected by a colorful neurologist in France.

JEAN-MARTIN CHARCOT

Jean-Martin Charcot (1835-1893) was a French neurologist and professor of anatomical pathology. He was the first to describe and to name multiple sclerosis and he also contributed to the study of a syndrome that he named Parkinson's disease. Of all the research discoveries attributed to him, he is best known for his research on hysteria and hypnosis. Charcot used hypnotism, which he adopted from Puységur's research, to treat the psychological disorder of hysteria. Hysteria was a mental disorder with physical manifestations including a wide range of symptoms beyond the patient's conscious awareness and control such as amnesia, anesthesia, aphonia,

51

abnormal gait, abdominal pain, blindness, deafness, paralysis and many other physical disabilities for which there was no organic cause. In addition to these psychosomatic illnesses were psychological manifestations of overwhelming fear, disassociation, multiple personality disorder, fugue, and a host of other mental symptoms. In public demonstrations, where he hypnotized persons in auditoriums, Charcot demonstrated that hysterical paralysis and mutism could be induced and removed under hypnotism. Charcot hypnotized his patients in order to induce and study their symptoms. He did not plan to cure them by hypnosis and in fact, he felt that only hysterics could be hypnotized.

Unwittingly he had tapped into the dark realm of the subconscious mind where deep hurts and scars of the past were stored but was unable to permanently resolve the inner conflicts. Fortunately a student, who sat briefly under Charcot's teaching, observed that hysteria was a neurosis caused by the existence of unconscious ideas.

SIGMUND FREUD

Sigmund Freud (1856-1939), who was born as Sigismund Freud but later changed his name to Sigmund, grew up in Vienna, Austria and became first a physician and later a doctor of psychiatry.

Early in his career he sat under the teaching of Charcot where he became interested in hypnosis as a cure for hysteria, believing that the symptoms were directly related to repressed psychological trauma. He observed Charcot placing a patient under hypnosis and temporarily removing the hysterical symptom. He was convinced the physical and psychological symptoms of hysteria were results of conflicts in the subconscious mind. For a time Freud used hypnosis in attempt to reach the subconscious conflicts. He soon abandoned hypnosis and formulated the practice of "*free association*," in an effort to reveal unconscious emotions. Freud believed that inner desires, secret wishes, and fears were kept in repression by the conscious mind. In psychological disorders, the unconscious efforts of repression caused too great a strain. Wishes and fears within the subconscious mind, receiving impetus from the libido, were exerting themselves into consciousness (cathexis) and another part of the psyche, which found these desires unacceptable, was exerting energy to suppress them from consciousness (anti-cathexis). The conscious mind found it too painful to allow the wishes and fears to surface and therefore refused to acknowledge the source of conflict. Freud knew the subconscious mind had to be entered in order to locate the conflict, and when hypnotism failed him, his theory of *"free association"* began to be utilized. Freud allowed the analysand (the patient) to *"free associate"* by speaking whatever thoughts came to the patient's mind. Any thought, or string of thoughts and ideas the previous thought had aroused, was to be followed, eventually leading to the real problem which was hidden from the consciousness of the analysand. In theory the conflict in time would be resolved.

Because of a low success rate, the expense and length of time necessary for therapy, psychoanalysis is practiced by few therapists today. It is no longer considered to be an efficacious therapeutic tool.

FRANCINE SHAPIRO;
EMDR AND THE TWENTY FIRST CENTURY

A more recent attempt to enter and reprogram the subconscious mind is a popular technique discovered by Francine Shapiro, PhD. As previously mentioned she is the discoverer of Eye Movement Desensitization and Reprocessing (EMDR). Dr. Shapiro was given the award for Distinguished Scientific Achievement in Psychology by the California Psychological Association and in 2002 the International Sigmund Freud Award for Psychotherapy presented by the City of Vienna in conjunction with the World Council for Psychotherapy.

The basic concept of EMDR, or Eye Movement Desensitization and Reprocessing, was accidentally discovered by Dr. Shapiro during a time of great stress in her life. She went for a walk to de-stress from her inner conflict and suddenly found herself moving her eyes rapidly back and forth. She noticed this rapid eye movement seemed to make her feel better. Further personal research led her to believe that rapid eye movement, which everyone experiences at different intervals while dreaming during a night of sleep, assisted the subconscious mind in reprocessing stress and conflicts. This research ultimately led to EMDR therapy.

In EMDR the individual develops a "target" prior to beginning the eye movements. A target is a snapshot image that represents the traumatic event and the disturbance associated with it. Using that image is a way to help the client focus on the event and a negative cognition is identified. The negative cognition is a negative idea about the self that feels especially true when the client focuses on the target image. The patient is asked to focus simultaneously on the image, the negative cognition, and the disturbing emotions and body sensations. The patient is then asked to follow a moving object with her/his eyes; the object moves alternately from side to side so that the client's eyes also move back and forth. After a set of eye movements, the client is asked to report briefly on what has surfaced; this may be a feeling, a physical sensation, an image, a memory, or a thought. The therapist then instructs the patient to focus on this thought or feeling, and then begins a new set of eye movements. Under certain conditions the therapist directs the client to focus on the original target memory. Periodically the therapist may query the client as to his current level of distress. The desensitization phase ends when the SUDS (Subjective Units of Disturbance Scale) has reached 0 or 1.

Although there has been some success with this technique, its success rate has been limited. Research is still in progress attempting to verify the efficiency of the method as well as how to improve it.

With all of the discoveries and therapeutic techniques discussed above, trauma, in the twenty first century, still remains one of the most treatment resistant psychological maladies on the planet. Scientists are still frantically searching for the answer.

The bottom line that remains is that somewhere in the inner mind the conflict still lives on. Mesmer, Puységur, Charcot, Freud, Shapiro, and others have tried to enter the dark world of the subconscious mind and enter the area of trauma. But there was a common denominator in which mesmerism, hypnotism, free association, and EMDR were all lacking. What might that missing denominator be?

The answer is quite simple — *none* of the above were states of trauma.

None of them shared the ability to open the door to heightened senses or heightened mental recording abilities.

None of them had the ability to actually change the physical neural pathways in the brain.

To access and discharge a traumatic memory, it is imperative that the sufferer actually enters a physical and psychological state of trauma. I am not referring to just the stress of remembering the event. I am referring to an actual physical and mental state of trauma. This would be a state similar to the state of consciousness in which the traumatic experience was first photographed within the vulnerable brain and then shelved away.

But what can facilitate this state of physical and mental trauma?

What can open the door to the mental mechanism that has the properties to heighten senses and heighten the mental recording ability?

What method can actually alter the physical neural pathways of memory?

In order to understand the answer, let us first study the problem in greater detail.

Chapter Four

The Nature of an Ancient Problem

The human race has developed in a world of uncertainties. Our early ancestors lived in a world much different from the world in which we live today. Children weren't taken to the zoo to see the animals — they were trying to avoid the animals in order to survive. It was a hostile world . . . a savage world . . . a world in which survival depended on ones ability to fight or to flee. Those that learned from prior threatening experiences were better enabled to survive future threats of the same nature. Those that didn't learn . . .those that didn't remember. . . didn't survive.

The human mind had been created with a very efficient mechanism that developed more proficiently with each surviving generation. Of course those in whom this mechanism was not proficient didn't survive and their nonproficient genes died with them. Those fincly honed for survival survived long enough to pass these genes on to their children; and their children to succeeding generations. This mechanism worked very well for our ancestors who lived in the jungles of the ancient world. Whether you believe our ancestors sprang from a proto-race of cave people or if you believe, as the author does, man was created by a divine Creator, the fact still remains that man lived in primitive, hostile surroundings, desert plains, forests, and jungles which necessitated the development and fine tuning of survival skills.

Picture a young man walking through the jungle for the first time on his own. He wanders far into an unknown area much different from the one his people occupy. As he goes deeper into the jungle, his senses record scents and sights unfamiliar to him. Perhaps the early morning dew carries the faint scent of a tiger whose protective coat of hair has absorbed the slight moisture of the morning. The young boy hears a rustle in the bushes. He hears a faint and unfamiliar growl. He turns and sees a beautiful orange tiger. In an instant the tiger leaps swiftly through the air, its heavy body slams the boy to the ground with a startling jolt. Claws gouge his flesh. Teeth sear his shoulder. The boy is terrified and frozen with fear. This is his first experience with this unexpected, unknown enemy and his immobilization is hardly conducive to survival.

Suddenly, from the brushy jungle pathway, warriors from his camp emerge with war cries and flying spears. The wounded tiger loosens his grip on the frightened boy and swiftly escapes into the jungle. The boy is brought back to the camp and nursed to health. Of course, his family explains to him the dangers of meeting a tiger. But something has happened on a deeper level. The boy, during the attack, was traumatized. During the state of trauma his senses were heightened. Somewhere deep within his physical brain an imprint was made. A picture of the scene was indelibly stamped in this imprint. The sights, smells, and other sensory messages were part of this imprint also. Like a DVD webcam recorder, everything was captured and recorded, stored in the virtual "DVD in the brain," downloaded, burned into the memory chip, and filed away in the boy's neurocomputer (the brain). The feeling of fear, anxiety, and heightened awareness was part of this virtual DVD.

The boy goes on with his life in the village. Of course this "DVD in the brain" of his traumatic experience could not continue to play over and over each day of his life. There are just too many other things in the course of an ordinary day that the conscious mind needs to be free to deal with. Therefore, the DVD lay mostly unplayed in the mind below the conscious level. We refer to this as the subconscious mind. The boy is unaware most of the time that the DVD is shelved there. The boy grows older and is now on his own. He is strolling through the jungle in search of fruit trees when he smells a faint whiff of tiger scent. Perhaps he hears a growl in the distance. Perhaps the area is similar to the habitat of the tiger he encountered years ago. Suddenly these "triggers" cause the virtual DVD in the brain to go into "play" mode and the stored program begins to replay part, or all, of the information back to the neurocomputer. His senses are heightened. He remembers the danger. He feels the danger. He experiences the urgency of the situation. Adrenalin pours into his blood. The boy at this point is charged with enough warning signals and chemical energy to either grab his sword and fight or, if he sensed the dangerous situation early enough, to flee away.

The terrible trauma previously experienced by the boy had proven to be very conducive to survival. The ability to store this traumatic incident in the brain, and the ability for outside signals to trigger such a powerful chemical reaction when facing a similar incident, was an inborn mechanism, an inherited trait, that allowed men and women to live in a hostile world and to produce children to carry on their lineage.

However, a young man who has returned from the jungles of Vietnam or from the deserts of Iraq, brings home trauma much different in content than those of an attacking tiger. An automobile backfiring and triggering the wartime "DVD in the brain" is hardly a mechanism for survival. Jumping into a ditch when a sonic boom is heard overhead, or leaping out of bed prepared to fight each time a door slams, is not an efficient survival technique. It now has acquired a new name. Clinically it is referred to as Post Traumatic Stress Disorder (PTSD). What was originally meant for survival has now become a disorder.

Let us now consider the general trauma induced by technological societies, followed by an observation of traumatic relationships within those societies.

GENERAL TRAUMA OF MODERN SOCIETY

Trauma served a purpose for the boy in the jungle. Future encounters with tigers could be anticipated in advance and his bloodstream flooded with the necessary chemicals enabling him to flee or to fight. However someone who is afraid to walk across a busy intersection when the light turns red because of a "DVD in the brain" has an inner mechanism that is a hindrance to modern living. The virtual DVD begins to play that awful accident in which her parents were killed and in which she was personally wounded. The sounds of automobile horns, motors running, brakes screeching . . . adrenaline pours into her blood to fight or to flee.

But there is nothing to fight or to flee from.

This is not the jungle.

This is technological society.

We were not developed to deal with artificial technological traumas. We cannot fight automobiles. We cannot flee from them. A really good example is to simply observe a dog chasing a car. Just what would the dog do if it ever caught the car? An instinct is at work here, but it is an instinct outdated in this modern society.

Trauma was meant to protect us, to save us.

We weren't built to endure the general trauma of the threat of nuclear war. We were not built to live in anxious fear of global warming and pollution, or knowing that they are slowly threatening the future of the earth. We were not meant to know in advance we were going to eventually die of a disease diagnosed by a doctor, or that the potential for that disease was inherited within our genes. We were not made to live in anxiety about how we were going to pay our taxes, make our house payment, budget our credit cards, or how to budget our income in such a way as to afford the rapidly rising price of gasoline. We were not made to worry about whether or not we were able to keep our job in order to feed ourselves and our family. We were made to go into the jungle and pick our food from the trees, berries from bushes, catch fish from the waters, or to till the ground and grow our food supply. Anxieties were concrete, physical realities — a tiger, a windstorm, a drought. We NEEDED the chemical release to enable us to stand against the tiger, to find shelter from the windstorm, and to search for and carry water from a distance during a drought. But how does one pick up a spear and fight inflation? How does one attack and pounce on the rising price of gasoline? How does one fight or flee the house and utility payments that a lost job can no longer pay for? We are experiencing stresses and traumas, with energizing chemicals flooding our bloodstream, and nothing we can attack. Some people succumb to their primitive nature, go berserk, and kill. Some lash out and become hostile and cynical toward others. Others learn coping techniques; some effective, others ineffective and even destructive.

INDIVIDUAL PHYSICAL AND PSYCHOLOGICAL TRAUMA

To cope with societal traumas many people become their own physician and attempt to buffer their trauma by self medicating with illegal drugs and alcohol. A self medicated father comes home late from a drunken spree at the local bar. He staggers in, shouting his frustrations at his small son Jimmy. Spewing obscenities and grating references to the worthlessness of the child, the father physically smites him. The child goes into a state of trauma. His senses heighten . . . everything in the incident is meticulously recorded in detail. The expression on his father's face . . . the smell of cigarette smoke and alcohol . . . the tone of voice . . . the scent of late night autumn breezes whipping through the doorway. The searing words, the degrading images the father is painted in the child's mind . . . a "virtual DVD in the brain" is created. A permanent specific trauma is forever ingrained somewhere deep in Jimmy's subconscious mind.

Of course Jimmy doesn't want to remember this incident every single day of his life. Perhaps he is even coaxed by his well meaning, but co-dependent, mother not to mention it to teachers or to friends, but to *just forget about it.*" The DVD program lies seemingly dormant in the hidden strata of the mind. Jimmy grows into an adult. He applies for a job with a good paying firm. As he sits in front of the interviewer, he begins to feel inadequate. Jimmy is not aware of it, but the interviewer's facial expression is reminiscent of that of his father. Perhaps the very position of authority the interviewer has relative to Jimmy, reminds him of his father's authority. Deep within his subconscious mind the DVD is triggered and begins to play. *"Jimmy, you are a worthless piece of trash that will never amount to anything! Can't you do anything right? You are worthless!"* As the message plays in the background of his mind, Jimmy has already decided he is not fit for this job. He will either sabotage this interview with his own inadequate answers or simply fail to follow up with the firm after the interview. Or perhaps the DVD began to play before he even went before the interviewer and he simply did not keep his appointment because he was convinced he *"couldn't do anything right."* He settles for a menial low paying job and barely makes it through life.

His father was better than he was. His father told him so. His conscious mind knew better, but his father was still speaking to him through his subconscious mind. Jimmy then begins to take on the characteristics of his father. His father was the authority. Taking on his father's traits means taking his father's position of authority and acquiring that same type of abusive power. Jimmy unconsciously becomes like the father he so detested. If you can't beat 'em, join 'em. Jimmy becomes an alcoholic. He comes home at night screaming obscenities at his small son and wife. And the trauma lives on to the next generation.

Instead of the above described scenario perhaps Jimmy will take the opposite route and, in an effort to keep from becoming his father, he becomes an overachiever, a workaholic, and his life ends with ulcers, high blood pressure, a neglected family, divorce, and a premature grave. In the end his life is just as extreme and dysfunctional as his father's life was.

A child molested by an offender is so traumatized by the event that it affects the rest of her/his life. Yet many succumb to the trauma and become sexual offenders themselves. They take on the persona of the one that was so powerful and exerted such control.

Some may form a reaction formation toward their abuser. This was Daddy. It isn't right to hate one's daddy. The subconscious then turns the energy of hatred into love. An abused daughter seeks *"Daddy"* in other men. She seeks to win *"Daddy's"* approval in the one she chooses as her mate.

A young woman molested, beaten, and verbally abused by *"Daddy"* eventually marries someone *"just like Daddy."* Of course she is not ultimately happy with her choice and ends up in a nasty divorce. She seeks out a new mate — and guess what? — He TOO is *"just like Daddy."* After multiple divorces she is stymied as to why she is attracted to and ends up marrying men that are just like the man she most despised and was abused by. She is being led not by rational choice but by a hidden trauma, or series of traumas, embedded deep within her psyche. Her past — not she herself — is in charge of making her present choices.

On the other hand she may become co-dependent, spending her entire life in the one abusive relationship that she feels she deserves and most probably is the only type of relationship she can feel comfortable in. She knows no other type of relationship. We are attracted to that to which we are accustomed to. We are resistant to change. We become comfortable with dysfunction, if dysfunction is all we have ever known. Anything else is alien. We fear the unknown. Our trauma centers are working hard to steer us toward survival. But we are no longer facing tigers. We are facing psychological dysfunctions our bewildered subconscious is trying in vain to protect us from. It is that very protective factor that is slowly destroying us.

THE ANATOMY OF TRAUMA

Trauma is the natural state of response to a threatening event. It becomes a disorder when psychological damage is impinged upon the psyche, adversely affecting an individual's ability to react responsibly toward reality. The event may be so disturbing that it changes the individual's world view and self image or produces confusion in these areas. It may affect their ability to cope with stresses of ordinary day to day living. The disorder actually causes physical changes within the brain, which results in a chemical imbalance of neurotransmitters, resulting in more stress and depression.

Such traumatic events may be one single event or a series of events. It may be the result of experiencing physical and emotional abuse or may consist of emotional abuse only. It overwhelms the person's ability to cope with the adverse event. It overwhelms their ability to integrate the emotions created by the experience and their ability to integrate the resulting thoughts into their previous belief system and world view.

There are eight traits commonly involved in the traumatizing experience:

1. Usually the trauma involves a violation of the individual's concept of human rights and the individual's place in her/his world view resulting in confusion and extreme insecurity.

2. It was unexpected.

3. The victim felt helpless in preventing it. The victim had no control.

4. It was emotionally overwhelming

5. The individual was unable or unprepared to cope with it.

6. It challenged the individual's self worth.

7. It violated trust issues.

8. It contains the fear that the threat still exists or a similar threat could occur in the future.

Trauma can result from a multitude of adverse experiences including physical abuse, sexual abuse, believing these abuses are going to occur or witnessing a sibling or parent being abused, verbal abuse (either a singular event or an ongoing series of events), invalidation, emotional abuse, rape, attempted rape, other types of assaults, automobile accidents, death, divorce, betrayal, combat in war, genocide, residing in a war zone, terrorist attacks, surviving acts of nature such as hurricanes, tornado's, earthquakes, tsunami's, drought, or even surviving a fatal disease such as cancer. Children may be traumatized by a parent or grandparent, by bullies at school, or molested by someone in authority in whom they trusted such as a daycare teacher, clergyman, a relative, or medical provider. Children are much more susceptible to developing disorders since they are so impressionable and have not yet developed a system of coping with various stresses. One may be traumatized by repeated experiences of rejection, feeling unloved, unnoticed, or being conceived as being different from everyone else.

Two people can experience the same stressful situation and one emerges unscathed and the other scarred with PTSD.

It is NOT the event that results in traumatic disorder.

It is the individuals SUBJECTIVE EXPERIENCE of the event.

It is her/his concept, understanding of, and inability to integrate and to accept the inevitable that results in traumatic disorder.

Some of the symptoms of trauma are anxiety, depression,

insomnia, nightmares, phobias, panic attacks, experiencing severe highs and lows, too emotionally responsive, inability to experience any emotion at all, disassociation, flashbacks of the disturbing event, feelings of inadequacy, low self esteem, and a host of other symptoms. One may not be able to remember the violation at all. Another may not be able to think of anything else. Months or years may pass without recalling it and suddenly something "triggers" the memory and one experiences a "flashback." Earlier we observed Robert who grew up in a dysfunctional family. The memories of growing up in this environment, and especially the situation in which he observed his mothers physical abuse one evening, resulted in Robert having life long bouts of depression. He related he could be fine one moment and then depression would fall like a dark cloud upon him.

You, the reader, may be able to relate to a memory that periodically resurfaces to haunt you or to disturb you. It may not have been something as drastic as a terrorist attack or living in a combat zone, but it may have been just enough to prevent you from living life to its optimal fullest. As a matter of fact, as pointed out in chapter one, it is almost IMPOSSIBLE for any human being to live in today's world and not have some measure of trauma hidden deep within them.

Whether the situation is a cataclysmic encounter or simple rejection from a loved one, the pain can become a stumbling block to releasing the real "YOU."

Antidepressants can alleviate the symptoms and help put one back on track but inevitably the pain will resurface.

How is this pain registered in the brain? No one is certain of the exact location where these memories are stored. One theory claims they are stored in a system that is reflected throughout the brain like a hologram, with one part containing the whole. Another theory claims they are stored in localized compartments in specific areas of the brain.

What we do know for certain is that a traumatic encounter is perceived acutely by the senses. You saw the attacker that leaped from the bushes. You got a glimpse of his face, the color of his shirt, and the surrounding scenery. You felt his arms clutch you. You smelled his cologne. You smell the flowers in the nearby flowerbed. All of the information that was rapidly gathered by your sensory organs was transmitted to a section of the brain called the thalamus and then filtered through the thalamus to the cortex and the amygdale. The amygdale is the "private alarm system" in the brain that goes off when any threat, real or perceived, is encountered. It is this part of the brain that attaches the emotional label *"fear"* and then transmits the warning signal to following five systems:

Memory Creation System: The amygdale transfers the warning signal of a threat and accompanying information to the hippocampus. The hippocampus produces words and labels for the emotional experience and will create the proper attitude toward the threatening event.
In the case of the above scenario an example would be, *"It is dangerous to be alone in this area at night. It is dangerous to walk near the bushes behind this building where someone may be hiding."*

Evaluation and Filing: The information and the memory created in the hippocampus is then transmitted to the cortex. The "headquarters" for this system resides primarily in the prefrontal cortex. The entire event is evaluated in comparison with the individual's world view, belief system, and her/his previous life experiences. When the threatening event is over, the cortex informs the amygdale and the event is placed in its proper file as a past experience.

Sympathetic Nervous System: The amygdale also sends information to the brain stem with the message that the hormone noradrenaline is to immediately be released into all of the body's organs to stimulate them into high gear in preparation to fight against the threat or to run for dear life. All the senses heighten, the mind is hyper-alert, the heart is pulsating faster in an attempt to supply the body with extra oxygen and energy for the battle or the retreat. The perspiration glands excrete sweat so that the attacker will have a slippery object that will be more difficult to hold onto. The vocal cords may be empowered to emit an involuntary piercing scream; an instinctual attempt to either scare the attacker or to alert others of the need of assistance in overcoming the attack. Or perhaps there may be some temporary physical immobilization to shield the organism from an unbearable source of pain. A state of hyper-alertness is accessed, not only to prepare for fight or flight, but to meticulously record every minute bit of information available to be later filed in "warning files" in case of future attacks. Other systems, such as hunger and sleep, are turned off so they will not interfere with hyper alertness.

70

Consciousness Circuits: The rational mind is taken out of "drive" and put into neutral gear. This is no time to try to rationally dissect or to analyze the situation. The instinctual consciousness goes into drive. The word "attack" is not thought. The feeling alone emerges and the action of fighting or fleeing simply takes place.

The Hormonal System: The information from the amygdale also is transferred to the hypothalamus (busy little amygdale we have). The hypothalamus activates a flow of hormonal secretion of cortisol, supplying the organism with an abundant supply of energy needed for the stressful encounter.

The Serotonin System: The hypothalamus transmits the information of the traumatic event to the raphe nucleus where there resides nerve cells containing serotonin. The serotonin is released to the cortex, hippocampus, amygdale, and all systems involved in stress response. Serotonin begins to turn down the alarming sirens of the warning system and returns the organism to a state of calmness.

Reevaluation and Final Refiling System:
The subconscious mind now begins its role as the caretaker of the files that the brain has created, adds the final touches, and carefully stores it away as a permanent memory.

There are four things that must exist in order for a traumatic memory to be created. One of these four will determine whether or not the trauma will become a post traumatic disorder.

As we have already seen, trauma is a necessary survival

mechanism inbred into our species. How does natural trauma become a post traumatic disorder?

First let us determine what is necessary to create the state of both natural trauma and a traumatic disorder.

FOUR CRITERIA FOR CREATING TRAUMA

1. A threatening event (actual or imagined).

2. A reaction to that event by experiencing it in an altered state of consciousness called "the state of trauma" in which all senses, conscious awareness, and mental recording abilities are excited, stressed, and heightened.

3. The presence of physical and/or emotional pain (emotional pain such as fear, embarrassment, etc.)

4. The inner labeling and the understanding of the history of that event, which is programmed into the stored memory of the trauma itself.

We can further condense the above four criteria, necessary to creating trauma, to:

1. The event.

2. The "state of trauma."

3. Pain.

4. Programmed understanding of the event.

Number one begins with the actual event. Whether real or imagined the event leaves a startling impression. A man jumps from behind a bush. You are frightened. It turns out to just be Uncle Harry up to his antics again. Although your senses may have been heightened to flee or fight, you soon discovered that there was no pain or threat of pain (number 3) nor did you enter in the programming data that this was a threatening situation (number 4). Therefore while you may remember this incident years later, you will most probably laugh about it. Or perhaps your inner mind recognized there was no label of "warning" or programming of a threatening event and therefore slowly deleted the information to the recycle bin as forgotten and unimportant trivia.

However consider a similar situation where a man jumps out of the bushes. You are frightened. This is NOT Uncle Harry. This is an unknown man. He is a rapist. Perhaps this is a mugging or an assault. You now have number 1 which is the event. Number 2 is the mental state in which all the senses become heightened and some remote part of your brain becomes a permanent recorder of every detail of the event. Number 3 includes pain (physical and/or emotional) and the "mental recorder" records the pain and/or threat of pain (something Uncle Harry's surprise attack lacked) in minute detail, etching the event into the traumatic memory. Number 4 is your understanding and labeling of the threatening event. You do not label it or record its history as *"A Prank by Uncle Harry."* You label it as *"An Attempted Rape by a Violent Stranger."* You write the history of the event into your inner program as *"a stranger, who is mean and violent, desires to hurt me, to kill me, he is more powerful than I. He is a man and men are not good. Being alone is not safe. Life is not safe. Life is full of fearful things."*

Or perhaps there may added shortly after the attack that *"I was dressed improperly, my clothing was too tight. I invited this attack."* Perhaps while still in a state of trauma an angry father shouted *"That's what happens when someone dresses like you do! I TRIED to warn you! Maybe you'll listen now!"* Or perhaps an insensitive police officer made an insinuation that you may have invited it. It may be that your father made such an insinuation about your way of dressing in the past and this shot through your mind during the attack and was programmed on your inner virtual DVD that you somehow were responsible for the attack.

In summery: You were attacked (the event), you went into a heightened state of awareness, in which a part of your mind became open and sensitive to recording every detail of the event. You experienced pain (emotional and/or physical). Finally, you labeled it as bad and why or how it occurred and what it meant to you.

It is largely dependent on number 4 whether or not you develop a disorder such as PTSD.

It is also largely number 4 which causes the DVD to continue to carry such a heavy charge of pain, fear, and traumatic disorder.

First of all, you CANNOT change the fact the event (number 1) occurred.

Secondly you CANNOT change the fact that you entered a state of heightened awareness (number 2) and that this event was recorded in the memory.

Thirdly you CANNOT change the fact that there was

pain (emotional and/or physical) involved (number 3).

HOWEVER you CAN . . . I repeat . . . you CAN change your programmed response (number 4) toward the traumatic situation!!!

You CAN release the pent up energy recorded and reserved in the virtual DVD.

You CAN break its tie to other roots of trauma and its debilitating effect on your life.

You CAN reprogram your virtual DVD, delete the title, rewrite your understanding of the history, release the energy of the pain, and refile it with the other memory files that are insignificant to your day to day function.

How can this be done?

The answer is so amazingly simple that it has evaded the scientific community for decades.

You must revisit the trauma.

You must FIND THAT DVD!

It is impossible to delete any information on the disk if you do not know where the disk is located. Remember that the disk player is hidden somewhere within the mind. Therefore in order to find the disk you must first TURN ON THE DVD PLAYER!

In other words, you must go into *the state of trauma.*

What? How is such a thing possible?

75

Very simple.

The answer is the ancient art and science of fasting.

Fasting can facilitate the state of physical and mental trauma.

Fasting *IS* a state of trauma.

Fasting can open the door to the mental mechanism that has the properties to heighten senses and heighten the mental recording ability.

Fasting can actually alter the physical neural pathways of memory.

Fasting affects the mental state of consciousness like no other method ever known to man.

What mesmerism, hypnotism, psychoanalysis, and even EMDR cannot produce, fasting can!

Lets us now explore how fasting produces a traumatic state and why nature has equipped it to do so.

Chapter five

An Ancient Answer

Our imaginary boy in the jungle had more to worry about then just tigers. That is one reason the tiger DVD had to be neatly tucked away in his subconscious until a trigger alerted the disk into play mode. There were other threats he had to survive. One of the most important threats to avoid was starvation.

For the sake of clarity let's give jungle boy a name.

How about Jay Boy?

Jay Boy has plenty of berries, fruits, and other sources of food to seek out for nutrition. Then one day he finds a drought has affected the food supply. Perhaps an insect invasion cleaned out an already sparse seasonal source. He may have wandered into an area that doesn't provide what his previous habitat provided. There are a multitude of scenarios in which Jay Boy could find himself without food.

His body sends a signal to all its cells, *"Prepare for famine."* His body enters a state of trauma in which all of his senses are heightened. Fasting heightens the senses. This has great survival value. He can now pick up scents that were previously unnoticed by him (Anyone who has fasted for any period of time can tell you that they can smell food a mile away while fasting!). This heightened sense of smell enables him to more efficiently track down a source of food. His sense of sight becomes sharper. Paradoxically he even seems to have more energy and to be more alert. He has been equipped by nature to access a state of heightened senses during a crisis. It isn't quite the recipe for survival to be moping around during a time of famine. Pig out on a big dinner and notice how all your senses are dulled. The senses are no longer needed in their heightened state. After a meal the body's energies begin to focus on rest and digestion.

Jay Boy finds different objects that may serve as food. He tries several which are inedible. Then he spies a berry he has never seen before. Cautiously he reaches out, plucks it, smells it, and, hoping it isn't poison, he eats it. Ordinarily this particular berry might have seemed quite bitter in comparison to the other berries he was accustomed to. However today this berry is the sweetest thing he has ever tasted. In his heightened state of awareness his subconscious DVD recorder is recording every detail. It is recording the area he found the berries in, what type of foliage grew in the areas that was conducive to the growth of the berries, the scent of the berries, and now the taste that has been registered as pleasurably sweet. When Jay Boy's season of famine passes, and he once more has plenty of food to sustain him, the traumatic memory is neatly tucked away until threatened again with famine. What he so laboriously learned by trial and error now becomes instinctual as his virtual DVD kicks in. It may have been very long ago that he discovered and ate the new type of berries that sustained him during his first experience of famine. But he cannot forget them. His DVD won't allow him to. He instinctively knows what habitat to migrate to. Triggers and cues in his subconscious will lead him to where the berries grow, or where the deer roam, or where the rabbit hibernates. It is a great survival mechanism.

Jay's forced fast has induced a state of trauma in which an indelible memory has been imprinted in his brain for future survival purposes.

For emphasis let me repeat; *Fasting is a state of trauma. Fasting allows one to access the subconscious mind.*

Something else happens to Jay Boy in time of famine. When the signal in his body announces, *"Prepare for famine,"* the cells in Jay's body rejuvenate and strengthen themselves in preparation to survive. Any damaged cells undergo autolysis. Cells ordinarily busy absorbing nutrition and reproducing themselves now shift into a state of self repair. The body fine tunes itself and the cells are revitalized. Neural pathways in the brain undergo repair, preparing the brain for optimum survival. Every bodily cell becomes strengthened and optimized.

Find it difficult to believe?

Jay Boy is not evidence enough?

Then let us explore studies done in strictly supervised scientific laboratories.

FASTING TRAUMATIZES PHYSICAL CELLS

Can fasting indeed facilitate the state of physical trauma?

A recent study indicates that fasting can indeed stress the body to the very cells themselves and stimulate them toward new activity.

An experiment, led by scientist Mark Mattson and his team at the National Institute on Aging, discovered that causing lab mice to fast every other day caused them to live MUCH longer and MUCH healthier lives. Mattson said, *"We think what happens is going without food imposes a mild stress on the cells, and cells respond by increasing their ability to cope with more severe stress."* He continues to say that perhaps it is similar to what takes place when you lift weights; You stress your muscles and they respond by growing stronger. [40]

So THAT'S what allowed Jay Boy to survive?

FASTING TRAUMA ALTERS BRAIN PATHWAYS

Can fasting actually alter the physical neural pathways of the brain?

Near the end of their scientific study they injected both the mice eating normal diet and those fasting every other day with a neurotoxin (kainite) that damages brain cells in the hippocampus, which is the area of the brain that is critical for learning and memory (the same area in which Alzheimer's disease damages human brains). They were shocked to discover that while the mice fed a normal diet suffered brain damage, the fasting mice were much more resistant to neurotoxin injury or death. They also discovered that fasting stimulated the brain cells to produce a protein called brain-derived neurotrophic factor (BDNF) that promotes nerve cell survival and growth. [41]

It had always been believed that once a brain cell was damaged or destroyed that it could never be replaced. However, recent studies conducted at the National Institute on Aging Gerontology Research Center and the John Hopkins University School of Medicine have shown that intermittent fasting not only increased resistance to disease and extended lifespan but also stimulated the production of new neurons! Fasting also was reported to enhance synaptic elasticity, probably increasing the ability for successful rewiring of the brain following brain injury. Again these benefits appear to result from cellular stress response similar in concept to muscular regeneration resulting from the stress of strenuous exercise. These studies indicate brain regeneration (neurogenesis) through fasting.

So we have found that the traumatic state of fasting both induces subconscious mechanisms as well as neurogenesis. A perfect combination for curing PTSD!

TRAUMA OF FASTING AND CHEMOTHERAPY

A study published in the Proceedings of the National Academy of Sciences reported that scientists tested the effects of fasting on mice, human, and cancer cells. Results suggested fasting induced a protective shield around healthy cells, allowing them to tolerate a much higher dose of chemotherapy. *"More importantly, we consistently showed that mice were highly protected while cancer cells remained sensitive,"* research scientist Valter Longo, PhD, of University of Southern California, said, *"If we get just a 10- to 20- fold differential toxicity with human metastatic cancers, all of a sudden it's a completely different game against cancer."* Stress that fasting subjected upon cells caused them to prepare for future stresses. [42]

SUMMERY OF ABOVE RESEARCH RESULTS

The state of fasting produces trauma. The subconscious mind responds to fasting trauma by turning on the trauma center's "virtual DVD recording" mechanism. The cells of the body respond to the trauma of fasting by shielding and strengthening the healthy cells in preparation for future traumas. Brain cells may also respond to trauma by stimulating new brain cells and probably promote the re-wiring of the brain due to brain injury. The trauma which induces these benefits is similar to the trauma our muscles experience when lifting weights.

It has been demonstrated by PET scans that PTSD upsets the chemical balance of neurotransmitters in the brain and may actually kill brain neurons. Fasting, however, is a trauma that repairs such damage.

THE MENTAL STATE OF TRAUMA

So fasting can repair neuronal damage done by trauma, but more importantly fasting can open the door to the mental mechanism that has the properties to heighten senses and heighten the mental recording ability.

Scientific research funded by the National Institutes of Health discovered fasting may stress us to a heightened state of motivation which nature intended to assist us in finding dinner instead of becoming dinner. When our bodies sense the stress of the fast and lack of caloric intake, levels of the hormone ghrelin are increased and secreted into our system. Ghrelin has been shown to alleviate depression as well as to increase sociability. The hormone increases the state of awareness.

Researchers believe that this trauma induced state of mind is an adaptive measure. The ability to find food in the wild requires intense concentration and clear headed perception. If hunger made man walk around in a daze he would likely become dinner for some other species. Heightened senses, which have been long reported by practitioners of fasting, have now been demonstrated in the laboratory. Hunger is not the only stressor that raises ghrelin levels. Ghrelin levels rose in lab mice when exposed to an older "bully" mouse and stayed high for several weeks. The threatening "bully mouse" and fasting from food, were both independent sources of trauma which effected the awareness centers. [43]

The measurement of ghrelin levels in this study have proven conclusively that fasting is indeed a state of trauma and a state in which a heightened awareness is induced.

Fasting can also increase the brain's abilities of learning and of recording memories. A study by Fontan-Lozano and colleagues (2007) revealed that fasting mice exhibited increased theta band activity in the hippocampus, the same area of the brain affected by traumatic events and disorders. Theta waves, beginning at 7-8 hertz, are the brain wave patterns the brain experiences at the deepest level of hypnotic induction in which, it is believed, the subconscious mind is tapped into. Learning is accelerated and the brain is more impressionable during theta band activity. Exploration of synaptic plasticity also revealed fasting mice exhibited enhanced paired pulse facilitation at the CA3-CA1 synapse. Fasting mice were quicker to learn and to create and file new memories. [44]

CLEANSING OF THE BRAIN, BODY, AND SPIRIT

Next we will learn that fasting also cleanses the brain for greater efficiency.

In the last century we have chemically defiled the waters, raped the land of it's valuable resources, and created a technological dragon that is exhaling it's toxic death into our atmosphere.

Our food supply has been generously saturated with preservatives, flavorings, colorings, stabilizers, and other man made chemical additives.

These toxins and chemicals are daily being absorbed into our organism. Over time these toxins slowly build up and accumulate in the tissues of the body and the tissues of the brain.

Fasting has been shown to cleanse the brain of these toxins which may also be a hindering factor in healing and rewiring of neural pathways.

It cleanses the body and the brain of toxins that have been accumulating in cellular tissue and in the microscopic tubes that carry vital elements to the brain.

84

The brain is made up of trillions and trillions of cells. Three thousand psychoactive chemicals interact within the brain which allows it to react to outside stimulus. More than fifty psychoactive substances have been identified that activate memory, calmness, aggression, and fear. The brain can perform over more than 100,000 chemical reactions per second. One hundred billion bits can be stored in the human memory, which are equal to over 500 hundred sets of encyclopedias! The brain contains 100 billion neurons and 100 trillion connectors just for the process of memory.

Within the physical brain, neuroglial cells supply essential elements to neurons. When neurons become damaged or die, they are consumed by neuroglial cells. Their function is to keep the brain clean and healthy. During the fast this function is accelerated.

Students at the University of Chicago fasted for seven days, which resulted in measurable increase of mental alertness and their progress in schoolwork was cited as *"remarkable."*

FASTING FACILITATES ACCESS TO HIDDEN EMOTIONS

It is no secret that fasting practitioners have consistently reported the fasting experience allows them to come to terms with emotional content they ordinarily were not in contact with. Fasting not only heightens sensory input from the outside world, but it also heightens perception of emotive content. Things that have been submerged in decades of mental junk are suddenly stripped of their veneer and the individual is forced to face his true feelings. This is why fasting has been advocated by the great religious leaders of the world. It cleanses the soul of obstacles standing in the way of purity of spirit and honest intentions.

One young man came to me announcing he was preparing to undertake a seven day fast. Having previously counseled this young man, I knew he was not proficiently prepared to face his demons from the past. He was not ready to see what was going to be unveiled within himself. I earnestly discouraged him from fasting. I reminded him that when Christ fasted he didn't see glory clouds and grand things. He saw Satan and was carried physically to a high pentacle where he was tempted. Fasting is not the reward — it is the battlefield. It wasn't until after the purging and trauma of his fast that Christ's miraculous ministry began. The young man was headstrong and began his fast against counsel. I met with him in the middle of his fast and observed his heightened emotional state. I observed feelings, conflicts, and memories of his past emerging more rapidly than he could cope with. I again strongly urged him to terminate his fast. He refused.

The next time I saw him he was confined in a mental institution. He barely recognized me when I went to visit him.

Fasting is serious business. Someone with severe emotional disturbances should be under strict supervision. Fasting is a powerful therapeutic tool when one educates her/himself about the method and it is used with reason. The fasting experience is not to be undertaken frivolously, but with much forethought, planning, and inner contemplation. Under proper circumstances fasting has been shown to alleviate mental illness more powerfully than any other method known to man. As previously mentioned Dr Alan Cott supervised many fasts and observed schizophrenia go into remission in a matter of days or weeks. Fasting had a normalizing effect on the imbalanced neurotransmitters in the brain.

This raises the question, *"Does emotional illness cause the chemical imbalance or does the chemical imbalance cause the emotional illness?"* It is sort of like asking, *"Which came first, the chicken or the egg?"*

I believe that there is a genetic predisposition in some people to respond poorly to certain stresses. They may have a borderline chemical imbalance when the trauma presents itself and the trauma sends the hereto unnoticed chemical imbalance over the line. Then again perhaps the individual had not yet learned effective coping skills when the trauma occurred and the impact of the trauma produced the chemical imbalance. It really doesn't matter because each disorder, both the trauma, the chemical imbalance, and insufficient coping skills, all feed off of each other and continually exacerbate the other.

PET scan images demonstrated that when one group of sufferers of Obsessive Compulsive Disorder (OCD) were given medication (SSRI's such as Zoloft or the tricyclic Anafranil) that the chemical imbalance in the brain was corrected and the OCD significantly diminished or went away. However another group in the same study was given no medication at all, but was given cognitive therapy and were taught skills which they used in preventing themselves from repeating the OCD behavior. After a period of time PET scans revealed that the chemical imbalances in this second group had also diminished or gone away. The conclusion was that with the correct skills one could alter her/his own brain chemistry just as effectively as medication could. It seems that chemical imbalances can indeed affect behavior AND that behavior can affect brain chemistry. [45]

The fasting method, which we will explain in the following chapters (6-9), involves both behavior and brain chemistry simultaneously.

FASTING RECHANNELS ENERGY SOURCES

During the state of fasting the energy reserves are no longer concerned with digestion, storing fat, being attractive to the opposite sex, having sex, or seeking out sexual encounters.

The body is alerted that famine has arrived and most of the body's energy reserves are redirected toward optimizing the organism for survival. We have already discovered the various functions that take place during the fast. Energy is directed to cellular repair, tissue repair, neuronal rewiring, toxic cleansing, autolysis, hormonal changes, sharpened awareness, etc. There exists only a limited amount of energy reserve for the organism to draw from and the fast is utilizing what it has. Anyone who has fasted can tell you the sexual drive virtually drops to zero during the fast. Of course it would — Jay Boy had no need to think of romance in time of famine! All that energy was redirected. Nature has much wisdom programmed into her.

What about the energy from the libido — that mysterious, powerful sexually based source of energy that is needed for the various mental mechanisms such as repression, cathexis and anti-cathexis conflicts, etc.? Sorry Jay Boy, but this is no time to worry about inner fears and wishes. You need all that energy to find food. You have either got to climb that fruit tree, catch that rabbit, or track down that deer. Unless Jay Boy was Hebrew, there was no manna in the wilderness for him. Any force of sexually based libido that was formerly engaged in guarding the subconscious and areas of trauma, must now let go of some of its former energy. Libido drops, sexual desire vanishes. Repression weakens. If Jay Boy wasn't so involved in finding food this would be an excellent time to tend to those tiger traumas!

You are not in the jungle. When you fast you do not need to search for food. When your libido wanes and repression weakens, your trauma centers are less guarded. The tiger is sleeping. What a convenient time to slip in and surprise him!

FASTING IS A STATE OF TRAUMA, THE DOOR TO SUBCONSCIOUS MEMORIES

So, in a final summarization, we have discovered that fasting induces a state of trauma, facilitates a state of heightened awareness, heightened senses, and heightened recording ability. We have discovered it optimizes the cells of both body and brain, repairs neurons, stimulates the growth of new brain cells, and is involved in rewiring the brain. We have discovered that it makes our emotions more accessible. More importantly, we have discovered that the subconscious mind and traumatic memories are much more accessible during the fasting state. For some these areas may be accessible for the first time in their entire life.

LIONS, TIGERS, AND BEARS, OH MY!!!

Theories have abounded and techniques created. New chemicals have been made and declared as the miracle cure one decade, only to be debunked the next.

The natural approach, one that has been prescribed for thousands of years, has been largely ignored.

CATCH THAT TIGER

The bottom line remains; somewhere in the jungles of the inner mind the tiger still lives on. Mesmer heard its growl, Puységur discovered its jungle home, Charcot entered it, and Freud met the "tiger" itself.

Modern psychological paradigms have taught us to accept the tiger, reject the tiger, medicate the tiger, understand the tiger, tame the tiger, or that the tiger doesn't really exist.

And the tiger sits back and laughs.

A TRIP TO THE JUNGLE

The only way to catch the tiger is to go to the jungle and re-experience the trauma.

But before entering the jungle you need a map and a guide. You need to know where to go and how to get there. Even more importantly you need to know how to catch that tiger lest you become like the proverbial dog we spoke of earlier, that chases a car and finally catches it.

We are just discovering how to do this. The only way to find the jungle is to enter the same state of mind you were in when you entered it the first time. The same door that was your entrance is the same door that is your exit. It has never been replaced. It never will be.

ALTERED STATE OF CONSCIOUSNESS

During the fasting experience, consciousness is altered in a beneficial way. During this state of consciousness the individual is able to access the hidden jungle in her/his subconscious mind. At first one hears the growling of the tiger. Soon one is face to face with the beast. It becomes just as vivid and lucid as the original experience. But there is one huge difference — you are now equipped with the tools to destroy the wild creature and lay it to rest.

In the next four chapters we will guide you through the method and tell you how.

Chapter 6

A Spring in the Desert

Let us now review in a nutshell what we have learned thus far, followed by a brief description of how an ancient method can be utilized in a modern world:

Traumatic memories have proven to be particularly resistant to both therapy and medication. Many types of therapeutic methods have been explored in attempt to reach the elusive memory that has been imprinted somewhere in the dark realms of the inner mind. Knowing that the trauma is hidden somewhere in the brain has given birth to various therapeutic attempts to immobilize it by slicing the brain, by shocking the brain, or by medicating it.

Other methods, such as hypnotism and psychoanalysis, have tried to reach the memory itself and discharge the emotional pain. These various techniques have been demonstrated to produce little or no results.

Every fresh new attempt has ultimately led back to a dry

and barren desert of lifeless, man made theories.

But beneath the soil of a seemingly useless wasteland, a spring of water flowed silently, patiently waiting to burst forth.

After many attempts, the prophetic voice of antiquity has finally made itself heard by the ears of modern science. It has at last burst forth freely, a refreshing fountain of truth, eager to quench the desire of thirsty minds too long parched by tradition — an effervescent spring in the desert.

You are about to discover a technique that has been with man since time immemorial, but has only recently been translated into the verbiage of modern science.

It is the technique of Fasting Induced Abreaction and Reprogramming.

The basic theory of this discovery reveals that during a traumatic event the human brain enters an altered state of consciousness which we refer to as *"the state of trauma."* In this altered state of consciousness, receptors of the organic brain are activated into a mode of acute receptivity and high definition recording. Details of the distressing experience are meticulously recorded and filed away in the subconscious mind until triggered by an outside source similar in content to the filed memory. As earlier noted, this is an inherited trait intended to facilitate survival.

To release the emotional charge of this distressing experience one must revisit the trauma. This has been known for some time, resulting in the above-mentioned therapies.

The problem with these other techniques is the fact that they are only REMEMBERING the troublesome event. One can remember a troublesome event as often as she/he wishes but that does not discharge it. One must not just "remember" she/he must actually ENTER THE STATE OF TRAUMA. The above-mentioned therapeutic approaches are NOT states of trauma — however, the fasting phenomenon IS.

Fasting induces the altered state of consciousness similar to the altered state of consciousness the mind was in when it first experienced and recorded the distressing encounter.

Also fasting allows previously inaccessible emotions to now be more accessible.

While in the traumatic state of fasting one begins to quiet her/himself by entering into contemplative prayer. Prayer has been shown to induce a beneficial state of consciousness. As soon as ones eyes are closed, the brain automatically begins to produce alpha waves. The longer the eyes are closed, the stronger these brain wave patterns become. Prayer takes one much deeper into this state. Studies have shown that prayer enhances a beneficial state of consciousness that not only deeply relaxes the mind but actually produces measurable chemical changes, both in the brain and in the body, which regenerate the entire system and enhance health and well being. Prayer warriors of all ages have known this and were aware of it before the first research scientist was ever born!

While in the state of fasting, and now in the state of prayer, one allows her/his mind to go to the trauma. The trauma is NOT remembered. The trauma is RELIVED. Fasting actually allows one to ENTER the memory and to relive it. This is a revivication of the experience. While in this state, all of the pain of the event is expressed. Tears may flow profusely. All the emotions originally felt will be expressed.

Anger toward someone in the memory, such as an abuser, may be expressed and shouted as the individual releases torrents of pent up anger. Great sorrow from losing a loved one may flood forth from somewhere deep within, or the individual may express tormenting guilt of having committed some wrong against another.

The emotion of the traumatic event is discharged and the area that the trauma previously occupied is replaced with— and reprogrammed with— a healthy view of the event which has already been explored and prechosen.

No chemicals, surgeries, or any unnatural methods are employed. Only the natural scientific art of fasting is utilized in retrieving, discharging, and reprogramming the traumatic memories and damaged emotions.

This is the technique of Fasting Induced Abreaction and Reprogramming (also known by the method's acronym as the FIAR fasting method).

A modern name for a very old method that was used by biblical prophets a long, long time ago.

Chapter Seven

GET READY:

The Terminology

Are you ready?

The question is NOT *"Are you curious?"*

The question is NOT *"Are you enthused to try something new?"*

The question is simply *"Are you ready?"*

Are you prepared to face your demons from the past? Are you ready to acknowledge hidden fears and wishes you have never acknowledged before? Are you ready to finally meet the real "YOU" without fear and with all openness and honesty?

If you are not ready for any of the above, then you are simply not ready to implement the FIAR fasting method nor to personally experience the results of the fasting phenomenon.

Scripture tells us that Christ was *"led"* of the Spirit *"into the wilderness."* (Matt. 4:1). The most important factor is whether or not you have been LED to fast. Notice also Christ was led there to specifically *"BE TEMPTED OF THE DEVIL."* So many have heard of the spiritual glories of fasting, that they enter it expecting to experience heavenly encounters. Not that this will never be part of the fasting experience, but we need to realize that we may very well be going *"into the wilderness to be tempted of the devil."* In the wilderness experience Christ met the devil head on and defeated him. Are you ready to wrestle with the demons of your past? Christ was tempted in his inner human desires . . . his appetite; vain spiritual glorification, power and riches of the kingdoms of the world. . . are you ready to wrestle with your most basic desires and inner wishes?

If indeed you are ready, then you are about to embark upon one of the most incredible journeys imaginable — the journey within.

NOTICE:

You may not initially find much interest in the rest of this chapter, and half of the following chapter, during your first reading. If so, simply glance through the following material and then skip ahead to page 105 and resume reading again beginning with the section titled, "Brief Description of the FIAR Fasting Method."

(If you have any difficulty with terminology, simply return back to this present chapter for the clear definition. If you do skip to page 105, PLEASE make sure you return to study the skipped material before attempting your journey via the FIAR method).

FIAR METHOD TERMS

The next two chapters will provide information needed to facilitate the method. It will be explained largely for the individual who wishes to use the method at home for spiritual growth. However, it will also be explained in simple clinical terms for the counselor who wishes to use the method in her/his private practice.

We should first define some terms we will be using:

Fasting: Abstinence from all food and nutrition for a predetermined period of time. Pure water alone is consumed.

Abreaction: Abreaction is a psychotherapeutic term for reliving an experience, a revivication of the memory, in order to purge and discharge it of its emotional content; a form of catharsis. It can also be a process for becoming conscious of repressed traumatic events.

Programming: The virtual "DVD in the brain" of a recorded event, or set of events, and the recorded understanding of that event. It is analogous to a program which is downloaded into a computer. Trauma causes a program to be downloaded into our neurocomputer.

Neurocomputer: The human brain.

Reprogramming: This term refers to erasure of an old programming and replacing it with a new one.

FIAR: Acronym for **F**asting **I**nduced **A**breaction and **R**eprogramming.

Fasting Induced Abreaction and Reprogramming:
The method in which fasting induces abreaction and the ability to reprogram the neurocomputer.

Session: The time we set aside to do the work on the damaged memory. This is done while fasting.

Negative belief programming : This is a negative belief you formed about the traumatic incident you experienced. This was programmed into the traumatic memory. It is a negative belief which is the root of your traumatic subjective experience.

Negative statement programming: This is the above negative belief programming condensed into a brief negative "statement." For example, *"I am no good."* There exists, somewhere in the background of our being, an emotional statement about who we are, and this is basically a summery of the larger belief history.

Positive belief programming: This is the new positive belief you will reprogram into the memory of the event.

Positive statement programming: This is the above positive belief condensed into a brief "statement."

Contemplation: Quiet prayer. Listening instead of a continued "yacking" to God.

Discharging the trauma: (See Abreaction above) Allowing the emotional energy and hurt to be released like steam from a pressurized steamer.

Reprogramming the trauma: (See Reprogramming. above) Replacing the old negative belief programming and the old negative statement programming with the new positive belief and positive statement programming.

Note: This book attempts to make the biblical art of fasting understood in scientific terms. The information presented is limited to the psychological and therapeutic benefits of fasting. This is not a theological treatise. Neither is it a science textbook. It is a simple guide for discharging trauma. Also remember that fasting and/or the FIAR method is simply a TOOL. When I state that *"one must enter the state of trauma"* in order to discharge a memory, I am speaking within realm of therapeutic paradigms. God can remove a lifetime of distress in but a moment! (One may also enter the powerful state in which your spirit, infused with the Holy Spirit, can take dominion and overcome any inner obstacles. I will revisit this subject in another book. Even then fasting may, or may not, be utilized).

Before proceeding to the next chapter please take note of the following:

Disclaimer:
The therapeutic techniques and the methods of fasting presented in this book are for educational purposes and the reader is instructed to consult her/his physician before attempting to utilize them. Expectant mothers should not attempt these fasts. Diabetics and those with a history of medical problems may need to begin with an essential diet for several weeks or months after which they may begin partial fasts and ultimately, with their physicians approval, begin to ease into the complete fast.

Although the author is convinced of the safety of the methods herein outlined, he must of necessity direct the reader to place responsibility upon her/his attending health care provider.

Chapter Eight

GET SET:

The Method

This chapter depicts the FIAR fasting method in an outline form, followed by a brief description of how it works. Familiarize yourself with this outline and then proceed to the full detailed version in the next chapter.

In this chapter you will first discover
I "THE NINE STEPS OF THE FIAR FASTING METHOD"

Next you will find an
II "OUTLINE OF THE FIAR FASTING METHOD"

This chapter will then conclude with a
III "BRIEF DESCRIPTION OF THE FIAR FASTING METHOD"

Then in the following chapter, chapter nine, you will finally be introduced to
IV "THE FULL VERSION OF THE FIAR FASTING METHOD"
(Please pay special attention to pages 119 to 126).

I

THE NINE STEPS OF
THE FIAR FASTING METHOD

1. MAKE SESSION PREPARATIONS

2. BEGIN THE FAST

3. IDENTIFY THE TRAUMA

4. BEGIN CONTEMPLATION

5. EXPLORE THE TRAUMA

6. DISCHARGE THE TRAUMA

7. REPROGRAM THE TRAUMA

8. TERMINATE THE FAST

9. CREATE A POST TREATMENT PLAN

The nine steps above are utilized in the fasting method.

A broader outline of the nine steps and the fasting method begins on the next page.

II

OUTLINE OF THE FIAR FASTING METHOD

1. MAKE SESSION PREPARATIONS

   a) Create a treatment plan

   b) Set the date the sessions will begin

   c) Choose a safe place for the sessions

   d) Prepare the environment for sessions

2. BEGIN THE FAST

   a) Pre-fast preparation

   b) The Fast

3. IDENTIFY THE TRAUMA

   a) Identify the traumatic memory

   b) Identify the "negative belief programming"

   c) Identify the "negative statement programming"

   d) Explore a "positive belief programming"

and a "positive statement programming"

4. BEGIN CONTEMPLATION

a) Center your mind and spirit

5. EXPLORE THE TRAUMA

a) Explore the trauma, the scene, the physical sensations, thoughts, memories, and emotions

b) Be honest, open, and trusting

6. DISCHARGE THE TRAUMA

a) Experience the memory and discharge the emotional energy

7. REPROGRAM THE TRAUMA

a) Re-evaluate the trauma and the "positive belief" and the "positive statement"

b) Reprogram the "positive belief" and the "positive statement" into the memory

c) Allow forgiveness and healing to take place and let the former memory go

d) Defragment

8. TERMINATE THE FAST

    a) Break the fast and begin post-fast diet

9. CREATE A POST TREATMENT PLAN

    a) Self educate

    b) Lifestyle changes

    c) Reinforcement

In chapter six was given a brief description of how the method works. The following is a brief description of how the procedure is performed.

III

BRIEF DESCRIPTION OF
THE FIAR FASTING METHOD:

You will first choose the date the fast is to begin. Next you locate a place in which you will feel safe and comfortable while doing the reprogramming.

You will prepare for the fast by eating fruit the night before so that it is the last meal residing in your intestinal tract, remaining there during the remainder of the fast. You will then begin the fast the following morning. You have planned to fast for three days. For three days you will be eating no food and drinking no liquids except for pure, clean water.

You will identify the traumatic memory you wish to work on. It may be guilt over some wrong you committed. Or it may be a wrong committed against you. We will use an example of a father in a rage screaming he was going to kill you because you were worthless and couldn't do anything right.

Prayerfully you will search for and identify the negative belief you formed about the event and which was programmed permanently into the memory (negative belief). To continue our example, you formed the belief that you were really worthless, you were unwanted in the world, you couldn't do anything right, and your father was correct because he was more powerful than you, smarter than you, bigger than you, and really intended to kill you.

Next you will identify a brief one sentence description (negative statement) about the above-mentioned negative belief. In our example it would most probably be, *"I am worthless!"* or *"I can't do anything right!"*

Now you explore a positive belief about the traumatic memory. In our example it may be, *"I am NOT unwanted in the world, I CAN do anything I set my mind to do or to accomplish, and my father was NOT correct, he is no longer more powerful than me, smarter than me, bigger than me, and he was not really going to kill me then and he surely CANNOT hurt me now!"*

Your positive statement, which is a condensed one sentence version of the belief, could be, *"I am NOT worthless — I am loved and worthy of love!"* or *"I can do anything I set my mind to do!"* You may prefer your positive statement to be a scripture such as, *"I can do all things through Christ which strengtheneth me!"* (Phil. 4:13).

On the second or third day of your fast you go to the safe place you have chosen. You will begin with prayer. You ask God to forgive you of any thing you have done wrong and ask him to protect you. You open your self up completely to him, be totally transparent and honest, and totally put your trust in him and in his care. Ask him to assist you with this traumatic memory, tell him you trust him with it and after the session it will all belong to him. Then you quietly listen to his voice. It may not come in words but you will feel reassurance and security.

After a period of quiet time you will, with eyes still closed, *allow* your mind to go to the traumatic memory. You will explore the memory. You will notice what you see there. You will recall the scents you smelled. You will remember the physical feelings. You will remember the emotions and thoughts you had. You will actually RELIVE the memory as though you were actually there. As a matter of fact a primitive part of your psyche will BELIEVE you are there. These are the natural mechanisms of the mind.

You will relive the memory from the beginning of the traumatic event completely to the end of it. As you experience it, buried emotions, wounds, and pains will emerge to the surface. These are feelings you have never adequately acknowledged and coped with. You allow yourself to weep. You may cry out for God to relieve your hurt. Or perhaps you may find yourself shouting at your abuser in anger. This is what we want to take place. We are discharging the emotive content. A buried anger toward your abuser emerges. Now you scream, *"I am angry at you!"* over and over at your abuser. You clench your fists and beat the floor. You may wish to scream into a pillow or into the open air. You scream until you feel the energy of the pain is discharged.

You go back to the beginning of the memory and relive it again from beginning to end, releasing all the negative emotion and pain just as you did the first time. You repeat this over and over again until you feel all of the negative emotional content is discharged. The experience has been similar to one many people experience when travailing and groaning in intense prayer. Perhaps those old time sawdust trail evangelists knew what they were doing after all!

With eyes still closed, you briefly rest as you regain your strength for the next phase. You will reevaluate the positive belief and the positive statement you previously chose. If it is still valid, you begin to announce the new positive programming into the memory. In our example you may shout, *"I am NOT worthless! I am loved!"* or the scripture you previously chose, *"I can do all things through Christ which strengtheneth me!"*(Phil. 4: 13). Let your statement penetrate to your very soul.

You will gather all of the possible energy and emotion you can possibly gather. With earnest intent and determination, you shout the new reprogramming statement over and over and over again. You will go to the beginning of the memory and as you relive it you will speak, shout, or cry the new reprogramming statement over and over. You will go to the beginning of the memory and do it again and again until you feel the new programming has registered.

With eyes still closed, you forgive your abuser and/or the

108

event. You gently let it go. Healing and feelings of freedom wash over you.

You have now deleted an old painful memory and reprogrammed it to never haunt you again.

You open your eyes. You slowly get up (if you were sitting) and stretch, yawn, and walk around your safe place. Go back to your contemplation, your quiet prayer and thank God for your deliverance. Tell him you are placing it in his hands forever. You forgive those that abused you and it is no longer your problem. It belongs to him and you trust him with it. Let it go. Next, with eyes still closed, quietly allow him to speak to your spirit. As he ministers to your spirit, your inner mind is deframenting the information change. Quietly allow him to speak. Slowly open your eyes.

Your FIAR fasting session is now over.

Spend the rest of the evening listening to inspiring music, or reading inspiring material.

At the appropriate time the fast is broken. You will take one ounce of freshly squeezed orange juice and one ounce of pure grape juice and mix it with two ounces of pure, clean water. You will sip this slowly.

You will have now completed an ancient method that contains powerful modern therapeutic benefits.

Congratulations.

You will rest better this night than you have in a long, long time.

Chapter Nine

Let's GO!!!

The Method in Full

THE FASTING INDUCED ABREACTION AND REPROGRAMMING METHOD

While the following may contain some material covered in chapter eight there is MUCH more material contained below that is essential for you to know. We will now begin with the first step and continue until the final step:

IV

FULL VERSION OF THE FIAR FASTING METHOD

1. MAKE SESSION PREPARATIONS

a) Create a treatment plan

Identify the possible traumatic memory. Plan out how

treatment will proceed. In a clinical setting the counselor will assist the client in formulating a treatment plan. The individual using the method for spiritual growth will need to create the plan through prayerful consideration.

b) Set the date the sessions will begin

Having identified the problem area, we now set a specific date on which to begin the fast. It is not to be chosen arbitrarily. You wouldn't want to begin your fast the week that Uncle Harry is coming to stay. He might jump out of the bushes again to scare you! You wouldn't want to schedule it when your daughter is having a sleep-over at your house for her birthday. Schedule a time when you know you can continue uninterrupted. Of course situations arise when family insist on planning something at the last moment, but this is when you put your foot down and let them know you have already scheduled the time slot in question and it cannot be changed.

Also if a specific date is not set, your subconscious mind WILL create reasons to procrastinate the event. Those hidden fears and wishes do not want to be disturbed or even discovered. You will unconsciously sabotage your own treatment plan.

Additionally you need to set a date so that you will know when to prepare for your fast.

Clinical setting: In a clinical setting the therapist should assist the client in choosing a date to begin treatment. Be aware that the client unconsciously sabotaging her/his own treatment plan is a reality and she/he may very well find multiple excuses as to why a date to begin cannot be set. This seemingly minor first step can actually be a major milestone.

Personal spiritual setting: For individuals executing the method for personal spiritual growth, you must keep in mind that there is an inner voice working against you. The tiger doesn't want to be roused. Be brave, be honest, be consistent, and like the commercial says, JUST DO IT!

c) Choose a safe place for the sessions

A "safe" place is somewhere in which you can be yourself and feel secure in being yourself. This may be your private bedroom, your computer room, a room in the basement, or if it not possible for you to have a place of privacy, you may wish to rent a cabin in the woods for a weekend. This should be a place where you know you will not be disturbed for any reason. This should be a place where you feel comfortable to vent pent up emotions through crying, pounding the floor, perhaps even shouting or screaming. This is going to be a very intimate and intense experience, and you need to feel that the place in which it takes place is safe for you.

d) Prepare the environment for sessions

Arrange for someone to run the errands you ordinarily have to run. Let those close to you know that this is a private sabbatical. If you are responsible for meal preparation at home, then prepare in advance something which can be stored in the refrigerator and which the family can help themselves to.

If you are on a short fast this may not be as important, but those on a longer fast may find themselves experiencing periods of crisis in which weakness or nausea occurs as a result of toxins and poisons that the fast is cleansing from the body. There may also be some measure of emotional crisis as feelings and conflicts from the past emerge. As mentioned previously it is important that you are in a place that feels safe to you.

Clinical setting: The therapist may wish to assist the client in determining whether or not she/he will be able to attend to certain duties and if and to whom these should be delegated to.

Personal spiritual setting: The individual may wish to simply set down with family members and explain that she/he is undertaking a fast. The scriptures do not prohibit revealing to someone that you are fasting. They prohibit you from standing on the streets and bragging about it as the Pharisees did. There is a big difference.

2. BEGIN THE FAST

a) Pre-fast preparation

It is of paramount importance that you know how to prepare your body for a fast. The ancient Hebrews knew how to prepare for and how to break a fast. If the last meal you eat before fasting is a Big Mac with cheese, please be advised that the Big Mac will most probably be in your stomach decaying during the whole time of your fast. During the fast you will not be consuming any further meals, therefore there will be no further meals to push the last meal you ate on through your intestinal tract. The Big Mac will simply lie in your stomach producing toxins that will in turn cause you headaches, weakness, horrible breath, nausea and a host of other problems. I often use the illustration that if I put an apple on one end of the table and a steak on the other end and left it there for several days, when we returned to the table days later, if forced to choose, which would you choose to eat? The answer is obvious . . . the apple. It may have browned a bit but it has not putrefied and gathered bacteria and even possibly maggots as the steak has. Food does the same thing in your stomach. Steak, Big Macs, etc. will lie there and putrefy producing toxins. Fruit however will not produce the toxic effect of other foods. It is important that your last meal before the fast be fruit AND PLENTY OF IT. The more, the better. If you are undertaking a longer fast, you will need to set aside the day prior to your fast to eat nothing but fruits all day. In the shorter fast eat nothing but fruits from noon until bedtime the day before the fast. Non-starchy vegetables can be used instead of fruits, but they have a less cleansing effect and produce a little less intestinal protection during the fast. All fruits and vegetables are to be fresh and non-processed. There are to be no additives such as sugar, salt, or coloring. If possible purchase organic fruits.

Clinical setting: The client should be able to follow this step without problem.

Personal spiritual setting: Scriptures tell us to ask God to *"feed me with food convenient for me"* (Prov. 30:8). Daniel fasted ten days on nothing but vegetable pulse. Wisdom would have us choose what would most benefit our bodies. *"Your body is the temple of the Holy Spirit"* (1 Cor. 6: 19).

b) The Fast

We have prepared for this day and at last we have arrived. Upon waking, the morning of the date you previously set aside, your fast will begin. From the time you wake up, until the termination of the fast, you will not eat any food whatsoever. One thing and one thing alone will be consumed by you . . . clean, pure water. Juice, pop, Kool Aid®, milk, tea, coffee, nor anything else is to enter your mouth. NOTHING is to enter your mouth but clean, pure water. You must not use chewing gum, breath mints, mouth wash — nothing! You should use a clean toothbrush WITHOUT toothpaste and brush your teeth using water. It would be very difficult not to swallow a minute amount of toothpaste in the brushing process. Also your cells are in a heightened state of receptivity and you will absorb toothpaste into your system through the skin, in the lining of your mouth. Any foods, calories, or substances of any kind will slow down and adversely affect the efficiency of the fast. There will not be much need for toothpaste anyway, because you will not be consuming any foodstuff or sugar. If you feel you must use something then use a bit of pure baking soda to brush your teeth with but THOROUGHLY rinse your mouth REPEATEDLY so that none of it remains to be swallowed.

Spring water or distilled water should be consumed. Tap water is a no-no. It contains chlorine and fluorides, the former being carcinogenic (cancer causing). It just adds more to the body's toxic load. Drink as much pure spring or distilled water as you desire. The water will expedite poisons being flushed from your system. Many people feel sluggish and out of touch with their emotions because of toxic overload. Once these toxins are removed they begin to think clearer and to be more in touch with themselves and their feelings.

Try not to be too active during your fast. You don't want to exhaust the energy reserves you need for tissue and neuronal repair.

NOTICE: *The length of the fast may vary between different individuals. Some may need to fast more days and others may need less. Usually two or three days is sufficient.*

3. IDENTIFY THE TRAUMA

a) Identify the traumatic memory

This first step consists of identifying which specific trauma is to be discharged. We are not looking for generalizations such as, *"I'm depressed because I grew up in a dysfunctional home."* Neither is the following statement considered to be specific; *"My father beat my mother all the time and it was horrible."* A targeted goal would be a specific traumatic event; *"I remember when my father came home drunk on Thanksgiving Day and beat my mother and threatened me."*

There may be many more incidences, but in this particular approach we will deal with one event at a time.

Clinical setting: In a clinical setting the therapist will assist the client in reviewing her/his history and in identifying the areas needed to be dealt with. Keep in mind that repression and avoidance may cause the client to steer away from the area needed to be addressed.

Personal spiritual setting: For individuals utilizing the method for personal spiritual growth; you may wish to include prayer. Ask God to reveal to you the areas needing tended to. Put your desires and fears on the alter and place your trust in a power higher than yourself. Only when you fully trust God, and believe him to be able to handle your fears and to understand your darkest wishes, can you discover where the tiger hides.

> b) Identify the "negative belief programming"

Identify the negative belief that you programmed into the memory. If an adult abused you and told you that you were worthless, you may have accepted that belief and made it part of the trauma program as well as a part of your life.

You may have been told you were going to be killed and you believed it.

You may have believed you were the cause of the family's dysfunction and the cause of them being unsuccessful.

In chapter eight we used the example of someone whose father screamed at them, threatening to kill them, and shouting how worthless the individual was. The individual's acceptance, and even additional guilt elements, became the individuals negative belief programming.

> c) Identify the "negative statement programming"

The above-mentioned example is the history, the story, and the detailed version of the belief. It explains why the person believes it and how it came about. However most of us do not go about day to day rehearsing the whole historical context of the trauma. There exists somewhere in the background of our being an emotional statement about who we are. If this statement is negative we call it the negative statement programming.

The negative statement is a condensed version or emotive title of the whole negative belief system.

The negative statement programming in the above described example would be, "I am worthless" or "I am worthless and deserve to die."

Once the negative belief and the negative statement are identified, we must then go to the next step which is to explore a POSITIVE belief and a POSITIVE statement with which to replace the negative ones with.

> d) Explore a "positive belief programming"
> and a "positive statement programming"

(Because it is essential to have some understanding of healthy thinking prior to exploring a positive programming, we will at present devote a little more time to this section).

In order to replace the negative belief and the negative statement, we must explore an alternative to replace it with that feels comfortable and true.

Often we carry the memory of the pain, believing it is a permanent result of an event long past.

Remember it was NOT the traumatic event or the crisis you experienced that created a trauma disorder and unhappiness.

IT WAS YOUR SUBJECTIVE EXPERIENCE!!!!!

It was your reaction to the threatening event.

Notice the three things below:

Event————Reaction————Inner Pain

The above left "Event" is the situation or the threatening event that you encountered.

To the far right is the "Inner Pain" or the trauma you experienced.

In the middle, between the Event and the Pain, is your "Reaction" to the Event.

Which caused your pain?

The Event?

Or the Reaction to the Event?

Let's say that the event is someone saying, *"I hate you!"*

Can those words actually travel from the speaker's mouth and physically assault you? Of course not!

So those words are not what is causing the pain.
It is your "Reaction" to the words that were spoken.

You cannot control the event but YOU CAN CONTROL YOUR REACTION to the event.

Let's imagine there is a knock on your door and there are people standing there with a large sign telling you that you are the winner of a ten million dollar sweepstakes. Can you imagine the incredible joy? Perhaps you would scream, jump up and down, or even faint. For the next few days you would be experiencing an ecstatic happiness that most people will never experience in a lifetime.

Then you get a telephone call that it was all just a prank.

From the time you were told you were the winner to just prior to the telephone call, you experienced a joy few people have the chance to ever know. Now had it NOT been a prank would the joy have been more? Would it have been less?

There would have been absolutely no difference at all in the level of joy experienced.

The joy came not from the physical money you were told you won, but from your REACTION to the belief that you had won.

The incredible joy came from you and you alone.

The joy ended NOT because you received the telephone call saying it was a prank. The joy ended because of your reaction to the telephone call.

If we could access that "reaction" ability and keep it perpetually divorced from the event situation, we could experience continual joy.

120

A thought can make you happy or unhappy.

You can choose to be happy ONLY if you have money. You can choose to be happy if you NEVER have much money. It is YOUR thought and it is YOUR choice.

While we may not always manage to feel like we have won the sweepstakes we CAN lesson the pain we experience by altering our reaction.

You can change your life by changing the way you think.

C.S. Lewis said, *"The heart never takes the place of the head: but it can, and should, obey it."*

We possess the power within us to form a functional or dysfunctional attitude toward any given situation or circumstance. Nothing on earth can change an individuals attitude except for the individual her/himself. This is the most important concept you will ever need to grasp. It is nothing short of a major revelation! It WILL change your life!

Chuck Swindoll wisely observed, *"The longer I live, the more I realize the impact of attitude on life. Attitude, to me, is more important than facts. It is more important than the past, than education, than money, than circumstances, than failures, than successes, than what other people think or say or do. It is more important than appearance, giftedness or skill. It will make or break a company . . . a church . . . a home.*

The remarkable thing is we have a choice every day regarding the attitude we will embrace for that day. We cannot change our past . . . we cannot change the fact that people will act in a certain way. We cannot change the inevitable. The only thing we can do is play on the one string we have, and that is our attitude. I am convinced that life is 10% what happens to me and 90 % how I react to it."

You and you alone are in charge of your decisions.

You and you alone are in charge of your thoughts.

You alone are in charge of your attitudes and the happiness in life that you do or do not have.

In the scriptures John the Baptist told Herod they could kill his body but they couldn't touch his soul. No matter what atrocities he faced, they could not put a finger on his inner self. Only HE could alter that. The apostle Paul faced starvation, imprisonment, beatings, shipwreck, and faced many other horrible situations but through it all retained an incredible inner happiness. Paul said, *"I have learned, whatsoever state I am in, therewith to be content."* His happiness was NOT winning a ten million dollar sweepstakes but it was in his salvation which was *"peace, and joy in the Holy Ghost."* Christ said that *"the Kingdom of God is WITHIN YOU!"*

There is no event that can force you to adopt an attitude that you do not choose to adopt. You not only have this innate ability, but you also have the ability to choose to increase this power, a hundred fold, by infusing your spirit with that of the higher power of the Creator. There exists much more substance than an abstract thought in the phrase *"nothing shall be impossible unto you."*

Victor Frankl, author of "Man's Search for Meaning," suffered horrific experiences as a concentration camp inmate during the Holocaust in Germany. During his suffering in the concentration camp he discovered the psychotherapeutic method of finding meaning in all forms of existence, even the most sordid and difficult ones, and thus a reason to continue living.

In the same manner, when we look inside the inner memory of some terrible thing done to us or experienced by us, we can choose to find meaning in it. We can choose to react positively to it. We can choose to interpret it in a meaningful light. We can choose to understand it differently than we were able to in the past when it first occurred.

Many, having never gone through a sordid event as described above, suffer not because the event is sordid but because of their interpretation of the event.

Many times our pain is COMPLETELY unnecessary because it stems from a warped view of the event. We may form a belief because of misunderstanding the event or we form a dysfunctional view of it.

This is the case in the majority of sufferers.

Always remember:

I AM RESPONSIBLE FOR CHOOSING
WHETHER I REACT RESPONSIBLY OR
IRRESPONSIBLY TOWARD REALITY.

As incredible as it may seem, we choose how we react toward any given situation. We choose how we view it and what we believe about it. The belief we choose may be the deciding factor as to whether the experience becomes a disorder or a learning experience.

Psychiatrist and discoverer of Reality Therapy, Dr. William Glasser M.D., once said, *"We may be up against a stone wall, but we don't have to bloody our heads against it unless we choose to."*

Every adverse experience is, should be, and can be a learning experience. Bad experiences not only have the potential to equip us with more efficient coping and survival techniques for the future, but they also have the potential to equip us with the tools with which we can reach out and help someone else who is struggling to make their way through life. Surviving a struggle with a tiger provides you with skills of how to avoid future tigers, how to survive an attack, or how to slay them. More importantly these skills can be handed down to your children. Each succeeding generation, adding to that vast accumulation of knowledge, becomes even more proficient in dealing with tigers. Thomas Edison was once asked by a young reporter how many unsuccessful attempts he had made in trying to invent the light bulb. Edison replied that it took him ten thousand attempts to make a light bulb that finally worked. The haughty, young reporter then laughed at Edison and said he must have surely felt like a complete failure. Edison shot back, *"Young man, why would I feel like a failure? I just discovered nine thousand, nine hundred, and ninety nine ways of how NOT to make a light bulb."*

When the first man strapped feathers on his arms and crashed in an attempt to fly, he learned how NOT to fly. His children disposed of the feathers, made a human kite, and after many cuts and bruises learned more ways of how NOT to fly. Eventually two men, who owned a bicycle shop, lifted from the ground and for twelve seconds actually flew twenty feet above an unknown, wind-swept beach called Kitty Hawk. Soon airplanes were flying from country to country and then one day a man set his foot upon the moon.

Many repeated failures can educate a society to success.

Many repeated failures can educate an individual to success.

There is pain in life. There is disappointment in life. But you can take a bad situation and discover a lesson that can enrich both your journey and that of others. You CAN take the lemons life gives you and make lemonade.

Positive growth from negative traumatic experiences was termed *"post-traumatic growth"* in 1996 by psychologists Richard Tedeschi and Lawrence G. Calhoun. They claim that trauma creates changes in how people think of themselves, their relationships with others, including the world around them, as well as resulting in profound philosophical, spiritual, or religious changes.

Calhoun and Tedeschi, who are also professors at the University of North Carolina in Charlotte, say trauma experiences can lead to growth, and have further discovered that *"reports of growth experiences in the aftermath of traumatic events far outnumber reports of psychiatric disorders."* They report these changes include *" . . . improved relationships, new possibilities for one's life, a greater appreciation for life, a greater sense of personal strength and spiritual development. There appears*

125

to be a basic paradox apprehended by trauma survivors who report these aspects of post-traumatic growth: Their losses have produced valuable gains . . . They also may find themselves becoming more comfortable with intimacy and having a greater sense of compassion for others who experience life difficulties."

They cautiously add, *"post-traumatic growth does not necessarily yield less emotional distress . . . post-traumatic growth occurs in the context of suffering and significant psychological struggle, and a focus on this growth should not come at the expense of empathy for the pain and suffering of trauma survivors. For most trauma survivors, post-traumatic growth and distress will coexist, and the growth emerges from the struggle with coping, not from the trauma itself."*

They again point out that *"there are also a significant number of people who experience little or no growth in their struggle with trauma."* [46]

It is this latter group that develops a disorder or troublesome and intruding memories from the past. The trick is to discharge the content of the latter *"post traumatic stress"* disorder and replace it with the formerly described *"post-traumatic growth"* belief.

Even the pain from the most horrific event can be altered. We must realize we DID survive, we are here, and the past is gone. I CANNOT change the event. I CANNOT change the fact that at that time I experienced pain. But I CAN change my attitude toward both the event and the former pain. I don't have to live in yesterday. Refuse to allow yesterday's misfortunes to be who you are today.

Explore the event, your reaction to the event, and the resulting pain. Reprogram the middle factor . . . your reaction. Remember that the present pain is nothing but a memory of a past event. All that really remains is your reaction and attitude. Explore a new attitude toward the event. Explore a new view. Explore a new history. Explore a new belief.

If that middle factor was *"worthlessness"* you can reprogram it to *"Worthy. I was in the wrong place at the wrong time but I am worthy."*

As mentioned before most of us do not go about day to day rehearsing the whole historical context of the trauma. There exists somewhere in the background of our being an emotional statement about who we are and we can program this statement with a positive statement programming.

The positive statement, the condensed version of the positive belief, is a very powerful seed to program into your mind.

The negative statement in the above-mentioned example was, *"I am worthless"* or *"I am worthless and deserve to die"* or *"I am worthless, I can't do anything right!"*

A positive statement to replace it with could be, *"I am worthy. I deserve to live!"* or *"I am NOT worthless! I am worthy of love!"* or the scripture we previously chose; *"I can do all things through Christ which strengtheneth me!"* (Phil. 4: 13) or *"I walk worthy of the Lord unto all pleasing!"* (Col. 1: 10). You may wish to select your scripture choice from a set of daily scripture reading cards, just make sure it feels right to you.

127

4. BEGIN CONTEMPLATION

a) Center your mind and spirit

Contemplation is simply a quiet meditative state of prayer. While the counselor may wish to employ a state using self imagery, the spiritually minded will wish to enter into heartfelt prayer.

Those of you seeking personal spiritual growth will enter into a quiet time of prayer. Simply close your eyes, think upon God, and speak to him as you would speak to your closest friend or confidante. Trust in him knowing he is good, all powerful, and understands every little feeling and every minute thought that has ever passed through your mind. Ask him to forgive you for anything you may have ever done wrong or anything you may have failed to do that you feel you should have done. Center your mind and spirit upon him. Forget everything else around you. Thoughts may attempt to distract you. You may be reminded of an errand you forgot to run, someone you forgot to call, a bill that needs paid . . . all of these distractions are nothing more than the growls of the tiger attempting to distract you and to discourage you from disturbing his jungle kingdom. Do NOT try to push these thoughts out of your mind. This will only cause you to focus upon them more. The thoughts will then rebel and become more insistent. When these thoughts come, realize they are not important for this "now moment" of your life. Do not give them attention. Let them go. Another thought comes. Let that thought also go and return your attention to the object of your prayer — God. Every time the thoughts come, let them go and return your attention to praying to God. Soon the thoughts will weaken in power and will go away. After awhile you may wish to stop talking to God, and to now allow him to talk to you. Keep your mind directed toward him as it was before, however now instead of speaking you are listening. His speaking to you may not come as words. It may come as a reassuring feeling. After spending some time being quiet, you will ask him to take you to the traumatic memory that has so disturbed your life. Go there. Do not be afraid. You are not alone this time. Go to the hurt. Go to the fear. Go to the pain. Go to the tiger.

5. EXPLORE THE TRAUMA

> a) Explore the trauma, the scene, the physical sensations, thoughts, memories, and emotions.

Go to the traumatic memory. This is a weed in your garden . . . a serpent in your Eden . . . a dysfunctional memory planted by the enemy. It resides in the dark, inaccessible part of your personality below your conscious level.

Within the mind is a structure of the psyche that contains all instinctual basic drives and no reasoning. Like a newborn baby crying to be fed, it has no idea where or how its meal comes to it — it simply demands to be fed. It makes no reasonable distinction between what is real and what isn't. This part of the mind believes the threat of the traumatic memory is still REAL. It is an actual threat. There is no difference between a memory and an actual event. This part of you will feel intense fear as you enter the memory. Know you are not alone. Enter bravely and prepare to face the enemy.

129

Find the memory. Allow your mind to gently hover over the memory. Observe it. Go to the beginning of the traumatic memory. Enter the memory. Be there. What do you see? Do you see the room, the hallway, the field, or the bushes? Do you see a face or faces? Look closely at the face. Do you recall scents such as cologne, a perfume, a salty ocean, or the breezes of an autumn night? What do you feel?

Allow yourself to feel the same emotion you felt when the event was real. Right now, this moment, this memory IS real for you. A part of your mind does not know the difference between a memory and an actual event. Take advantage of this and experience the memory in every detail. What thoughts are going through your mind? What "self talk" dialogues are you engaged in? What fleeting thoughts shoot through your mind? Do not stop them. Do not resist them. These are YOUR thoughts. Some of these thoughts may have been fed to you from an outside source, but it was you who ultimately accepted them. This does not make you good or bad. This "just is." What are you feeling physically? Do you feel the floor or ground below your feet? Do you feel the hands of your abuser? The memory is there. The feeling is there. It is all recorded. If you do not feel your abusers hands, it is because some mechanism of repression and fear is hiding it from you. Go ahead and feel the sensations, the pain, the fear, and the somatic. It is all right. It is not an act of sin to recall it. It is not a "fantasy" of aggression or pleasure. It is a memory that is already there, and you are simply bringing it forth in order to discharge the negative energy it contains. You are not going to linger in it. You are not going to savor it. You are going to dispose of it.

a) Be honest, open, and trusting.

Remember: Be completely open, be innocent, and be honest. Shakespeare created Hamlets quote, *"Above all else, to thine own self be true."* You may lie to your friends, you may lie to your family, you may lie to all of the world, but whatever you do, do NOT lie to yourself. Do NOT lie to God. An addict lies to everyone around them by denying they have a problem. But when that addict lies to her/himself . . . the addict is beyond help. The great psychologist Carl Rogers once said, *"The curious paradox is that when I accept myself just as I am, then I can change."*

6. DISCHARGE THE TRAUMA

a) Experience the memory and discharge
the emotional energy

You have successfully entered the memory of the trauma. Go to the beginning of it. Let the DVD in your brain play as though you are actually there. Again remember a part of you, not knowing the difference between reality and a memory, actually believes you ARE there. This is the Id. This is the child within you. This is the "Little Jimmy," not James the adult. This is "Little Patty" or "Little Becky," not Patricia the adult or Rebecca the adult. "Little Patty" is still in there somewhere. She is frightened and alone. She is hurting. She has been waiting for someone to rescue her. The time for redemption has arrived. "Little Patty" is about to go free. BECOME that child or that person at the age you were when you were wounded. Feel the pain and unfairness. Feel the physical sensations. Feel the inner turmoil and anger. FEEL IT. Go ahead and cry. Do not hold back the tears. Let "little Patty" or "little Jimmy" weep. Stay with the feeling. Stay with the pain. Do not attempt to analyze it or to understand it. Do not rationalize whether you were right or wrong, or whether the incident was, or was not, as bad as you thought it was. Experience it as if it were in "the now" moment.

Next you will do something you may not have been able to do in the original experience. You will now announce your feelings out loud. Address the remembered abuser. Say exactly what you feel. Shout it. Scream it. *"I am hurt! You hurt me!" or "You violated me!" or "I am afraid!"* If anger and hatred is there, do not be afraid to express it. Remember you are NOT inserting a new program into the memory. You are DELETING an old one. It is not a sinful act if you shout, *"I feel hate toward you!"* You are not creating a new hate, but you are releasing the energies of an old one that was already there. Look at the one that violated you and scream, *"I hate what you did to me! You hurt me!"* Allow the anger, the hurt, the guilt, and the pain to rise to the surface. You may take your pain to God, crying out,*"God, please take the hurt from me!"* Express yourself with abandoned emotion. Scream out from your innermost being. Scream out your emotion over and over and over again, until it is drained. You may wish to scream into a pillow or to shout into the air. You may need to clench your fists and beat the floor. Say what you feel and feel what you say.

Next go back to the beginning of the memory and go through it again. Relive it in all of its intensity. When you get to the end of the memory return AGAIN to the beginning and go through it to the end. Do this over and over again until it is completely drained of all of its emo-

132

tional and threatening energy.

7. REPROGRAM THE TRAUMA

a) Re-evaluate the trauma and the "positive belief " and the "positive statement"

b) Reprogram the "positive belief " and the "positive statement" into the memory

Stay in the memory. Re-evaluate the positive belief you previously chose. If it does not feel appropriate, choose another belief that is appropriate. Go to the beginning of the memory and announce the positive belief. For example the old negative belief may have been, *"Everything I do turns out wrong. I am no good. I am a burden to the rest of the family. I am a worthless person because I do everything wrong. I will never amount to anything or succeed in life."* The NEW positive belief to replace it with would be, *"Everything I do does NOT turn out wrong. I AM a good person. My father was an abusive alcoholic and took his anger out on me. I WILL amount to something. I WILL succeed. I AM A CHILD OF GOD! I am a royal member of his Kingdom! I am a good person!"*

The condensed negative statement of the above negative belief could have been, *"You can't do anything right!"*

A scripture or a condensed phrase of the above positive belief could be one of those we previously chose, *"I am NOT worthless! I am worthy of love!"* or *"I can do all things through Christ which strengtheneth me!"* (Phil. 4: 13).

The negative belief is the belief you unconsciously chose to accept about the memory. The negative statement, the condensed phrase that briefly sums up the belief in a few short words, is more powerful, just as condensed milk is richer than ordinary milk. The statement runs quietly in the background of our neurocomputer in the same manner that the Windows Vista® program runs in the background of your PC. It is an emotional statement about who we are.

Another example of both a belief and a statement programming would be that of a young child that may have been repeatedly sexually molested by an adult. Perhaps over months or years of this behavior the child realizes the act stroking certain body parts actually produced a pleasurable sensation and the child may have, on occasion, even approached the adult to experience it again. Or perhaps the child was flirtatious with the adult in an attempt to gain the love the child was lacking in her/his life. In this situation the negative belief, corroded with guilt, may have been, *"I brought the sexual abuse upon myself. Sometimes I even enjoyed it. I am no good. It's my fault."* The positive belief programming to replace it with could be, *"I did NOT bring this upon myself! I was too young to protect myself from an overpowering adult! My body felt pleasure only because it was meant to feel pleasure from stimulation. You knew better. You took advantage of me. I did not create the situation. You created a situation that caused me to fill my mind with guilt! I am now choosing to no longer be under bondage to you in the belief that I caused this to happen!"* The condensed positive statement of the above new belief could be, *"I did NOT bring this upon myself!"* Revisit the memory and reprogram the statement into the memory. This will become the new emotional statement that will now be running somewhere in the background of your being.

As you experience the memory again announce the new positive statement reprogramming phrase. In the first example it would, again, be the pre-chosen scripture, *"I CAN do ALL things through Christ that strengtheneth me!"* (Phil. 4:13) or in the second example, *"I did NOT bring this upon myself "* with all the intensity and emotion you can muster. When you become exhausted rest for a few moments, but do not open your eyes or leave the memory. Take a few deep breathes. Tense every muscle in your body, build up all the emotion humanly possible, build up all the energy available, and from deep within you, with all the determination and feeling you possess, repeat your reprogramming scripture or phrase with utmost intensity. Then go to the beginning of the memory and reprogram it again. Do this over and over again until you feel the new reprogramming has been permanently imprinted in the memory.

Again, just as you did when discharging the memory, repeat it from deep within you. THIS time you are NOT discharging old content, but you are imprinting and RECORDING new content. Scream with all of the intensity you can feel. Do not scream to just be screaming, but scream out from your inner emotional reserves over and over and over again until it is drained. You may wish to scream into a pillow or to shout into the air. You may need to clench your fists and beat the floor. You may need to stomp your feet. You may need to weep and to cry out the statement. Say it with feeling. You must believe it! You must MEAN it!!!

Next go back to the beginning of the memory and go through it again. Reprogram the new statement into the memory with the greatest of intensity. When you get to the end of the memory, return AGAIN to the beginning and go through it to the end. Do this over and over again until you feel it has been completely reprogrammed.

c) Allow forgiveness and healing to take place and let the former memory go

With eyes remaining closed, forgive your abuser or abusers, and even the event itself. Next, eyes still closed, enter into contemplative prayer again. Take this memory, give it to God, and then forever let it go.

While it may seem difficult, you may be surprised how easily this next process may flow. You have already purged and replaced the territory with a new foundation. You successfully entered the hidden jungle of your tormenting pain, faced the tiger, defeated him, and replaced him with a sleeping kitty. The tiger and his former power is no more. It will never be again. It has been refiled as an old memory only. It is no longer a living event that continues to live somewhere inside of you. The living event has been refiled as an inert memory and a new title has replaced the name on the new file with a new understanding of the event. You have arrived to a place long overdo. It is called "closure." You may now, at last, forgive the tiger. You may, at last, forgive the previously tormenting event. At long last you may simply and permanently let it go. Your heart, mind, soul, and spirit is receiving healing from the powerful force we call forgiveness.

When my son was a little boy, he one day asked me to take him to the park to fly a kite. He was inexperienced at that early age with kite flying but insisted he do it himself. He grabbed the kite and threw it at the wind. It immediately crashed to the ground. Frustrated he picked it up again and thrust it toward the sky in an effort to force the kite to fly. Again it crashed. I taught him something that day that he was to never forget. Although the wind was right and the kite was ready, he just could not force the kite to fly — he had to let it go.

Let it go.

Let go of the pain, the memory, the person or persons, and let your former feelings toward the person, or persons, go. Forgive and let go. Give it all to God. Trust him with it. Put it into his hands. You may be amazed at the flow of freedom you will experience as you simply forgive and at long last just forever *let it go.*

Let healing, forgiveness, and love freely flow through your mind and heart. Accept the freedom and joy that is yours to experience. You will never be the same again.

d) Defragment

When deleting an old program from the computer, it sometimes leaves bits and pieces of the old registry behind that must be cleaned up with a registry cleaner. It also creates fragmented files within the system that have to be rearranged, defragmented, and refiled.

You have deleted an old program from your inner mind. If stray fragments of the old registry show up from time to time, simply clean the registry, defragment, and refile by repeating the discharging and reprogramming phases.

After your original session, you have deleted an old program, and now you must optimize by an initial defragmentation. Simply open your eyes. Stretch, yawn, walk around the session room a bit, and take a few deep breathes. Next enter the state of contemplative and quiet prayer. Address the Lord and ask him to continue to keep you safe within his care. Pause and listen to his voice. As you quiet yourself and experience his joy, you will slowly defragment the session within both your inner mind and in your spirit. Open your eyes. After leaving the session room, you should continue to spend some quiet time in some private activity you find pleasurable. It may be reading a good book, listening to music, or enjoying an inspirational program.

8. TERMINATE THE FAST

a) Break the fast and begin post-fast diet

The first thing one should break the fast on is fruit juice. The digestive system has been in the state of hibernation during the extent of the fast and should not be suddenly "jolted" back into the anabolic stage suddenly. Also you do not want to cause your system to have to ram the breaks, shift gears, and go into the metabolic state of intense digestion. Your system still needs energy directed toward healing the neurons in the brain and for rewiring synaptic paths that have been changed during reprogramming. The best thing to break a fast on is the following: One ounce of freshly squeezed orange juice, one ounce of pure grape juice, and two ounces of pure, clean water mixed together. This mixture of one part juice diluted with one part water, would seem bland any other time. You will be surprised how absolutely delicious it will taste after a fast!

Remember that your body has been deprived of nutrition for some time now. Your digestion system has also been optimized in preparation for the time in which food would be found and consumed. Your body is prepared to make the most use out of what it will receive. For example, if you ate a hot dog on an ordinary day, you would consume the calories, fat, sugar, additives, and other content of the hot dog, of which some of this content would be automatically used by your general body metabolism, some of the content of the hot dog would pass undigested through the intestinal system (an even greater amount of fats and calories may be rushed out of the system if sufficient fiber has been ingested), and some of the calories would go to specific organs of the body to be used as fuel, leaving the extra calories to be stored in the fat reserves. However, after the fast, your digestion system has now been optimized. In the optimized post fasting digestive system 100 PER CENT OF THE FOOD THAT IS CONSUMED, IS ABSORBED BY THE HUNGRY ORGANS OF THE BODY!!!

Think of a sponge soaked in a cup of ordinary water. Remove it. Dip that same sponge into a second cup of water that is mixed with red dye. Let it set a moment, and take it out. The sponge has absorbed some of the red dye water—but not much! It had already absorbed an efficient amount of regular water from the first cup.

Now take a sponge in which ALL THE WATER has been squeezed out. Dip that sponge into the water of red dye. Let it set a moment and take it out. Did it absorb more red dye water than the previous sponge? OF COURSE! It absorbed ALL THE WATER it could possibly absorb. The latter sponge was a "hungry" sponge.

Before the fast you were like the first sponge. Your body took what it needed and that was it. After the fast your body was like the squeezed out sponge and your body ABSORBED 100 PER CENT OF EVERYTHING IT CONSUMED!!!

Would you seriously like for your body to 100 per cent consume a Big Mac and send 100 per cent of that greasy, artery clogging, cancer cell producing fat to your arteries and organs? Would you seriously want to intentionally send all the preservatives, colorings, flavorings, and cancer producing nitrate in that hot dog to every single veraciously hungry cell in your body? If not then you should rule out Big Macs and hot dogs as food with which to terminate a fast.

As a matter of fact, you will not be returning to ordinary eating for as many days as you fasted. In other words if you fasted two days it will take two days to properly break your fast and return to a normal diet. If you fasted ten days, it will take ten days to properly break your fast and return to normal eating. To do otherwise would be to ruin many of the great benefits received from the fast.

If you have fasted for three days, you may wish to break your fast late in the evening, the third day before retiring to bed. For example if your fast began after 10:30 PM on Monday, it will be exactly three days after 10:30 PM on Thursday, which is the third day of your fast (a total of three twenty four hour days). The benefit of breaking your fast by drinking this juice before bedtime is the fact that your newly awakened digestive system, and its accompanying appetite, will have to sleep until morning. You have now slept through the most aggressive portion of hunger rebound. The following is based upon a fast of

140

only two or three days: The next morning, after breaking the fast on the diluted juice, eat a light breakfast of fruits. At lunch add vegetables. At supper add carbohydrates such as bread or cereal and some fresh yogurt or other dairy product. The next day continue eating increasingly larger portions of food, eventually adding proteins such as fish or chicken. The third day you may resume normal eating. If you still have a voracious appetite CONTROL IT until it once again becomes normal. It takes much more self control AFTER a fast than during one. This will strengthen your abilities of controlling the flesh and the self.

9. CREATE A POST TREATMENT PLAN

a) Self Educate

Arm yourself with inspirational books and tapes. Educate yourself about trauma and healthy mental attitudes. One book I highly recommend is "Healing for Damaged Emotions," by David A. Seamonds. I have seen virtual miracles take place in the lives of people I have recommended this book to. Another good book by the same author is, "Healing for Damaged Memories". More beneficial reading can be derived from the book "Reality Therapy," by Dr. William Glasser M.D. If you suffer from Obsessive Compulsive Disorder, I recommend you add "Brain Lock," by Dr. Jeffrey Schwartz M.D., to your list. Even if you do not have OCD, you will glean a wealth of information from the book. Read, read, and re-read the profound, mentally healthy, jewels of wisdom in the New Testament book of Matthew 6: 19 to 7: 12. Ponder on it. Memorize portions of it or perhaps all of it. Let the words and message sink deep within you.

Educate yourself with new coping techniques and living skills. Many people often wander throughout life making poor decisions and reaping poor results because the only tools they were equipped with were those learned in a dysfunctional situation. Abraham Maslow said, *"When the only tool you have is a hammer, all problems begin to resemble nails."*

b) Lifestyle changes

I would suggest you not return to your old eating habits. I promise you that you that your doctor will never diagnose you with a *"hamburger"* deficiency, a *"hot dog deficiency,"* or a *"cake and pie deficiency."* Your body was not created to consume such non-foods and you will fare much better, both mentally and physically, without them.

Start an exercise program of daily fast paced walking.

Take vitamins and minerals and especially boost your vitamin E and C intake. I personally take no less than 400 IU of vitamin E and 500 MG. of C each day. Take a daily multiple vitamin that has a good range of all of the essential vitamins. However, I must caution you to be aware of effects from multiple vitamins containing high doses of B vitamins. While they may be beneficial in supplying the body with more energy, I have observed that, quite often, too high a dosage of B vitamins can overly stimulate the appetite resulting in weight gain. Unless you desire a weight gain, you may wish to choose a multiple vitamin that is lower in B vitamins (and just to be safe, continue to watch for any increases in appetite). Gotu Kola and Ginseng are excellent herbal supplements. For continued mental and emotional well being,

142

take SAINT JOHNS WORT and take it EVERY DAY. This herb is the natural Prozac of the nutritional world. It has been demonstrated to assist balancing the neuro-transmitters in the brain that are responsible for good mental health and emotional well being. It has been studied in research labs and shown to be effective in alleviating depression and anxiety. It also assists in resisting the stresses of traumatic memories and equips the brain to be more resistant in producing a Post Traumatic Stress Disorder. It also is involved in neurogenesis, which is the production of new brain cells, due to its SSRI-like abilities.

I would caution you to speak to your doctor before adding any of these supplements to your diet or even before implementing a fast. Saint Johns Wort may boost the effects of antidepressants such as Zoloft, Prozac, etc., which could be dangerous for those already on a high antidepressant dosage. Saint Johns Wort can also make one more sensitive to the sun, so you may need to be more cognizant of wearing sunscreen and sunglasses, which you should be wearing anyway. The damage modern technology has inflicted upon the ozone layer is allowing more damaging ultra violet radiation to infiltrate our atmosphere than our bodies were created to withstand.

In summery, you would greatly benefit from an increased dose of vitamins E and C, possibly a multivitamin, Gotu Kola, Ginseng, and MOST importantly Saint Johns Wort.

c) Reinforcement

We are creatures of habit.

Once a habit is established, good or bad, it is always easier to take the path of least resistance and continue performing the old habit.

We may have established an "emotional habit" of feeling a certain way. Growing in a dysfunctional home, we may have faced emotional turmoil every single day of our lives. To not experience the turmoil and the drama of dysfunction may cause one to feel out of his comfort zone. You may find it easier to slip back into the "emotional habit" of feeling turmoil, depression, and constant drama.

It takes twenty one days to establish a new habit. For twenty one days after your therapeutic fasting session, continue to drill your new belief and positive statement into your soul. Type out your positive statement on paper and tape it to your bathroom mirror, your refrigerator, and in your car. Find scriptures relating to your positive statement. Memorize them. Every morning establish the habit of a quiet time in prayer, and scripture reading, and continue it beyond the twenty one day period of time you have devoted to changing old habits and continue it for the rest of your life. Every day will be started with the charge of positive energy and spiritual rejuvenation.

Connect with a good support group. Gather positive people around you . Be faithful to your church and other support groups. Devote time to HELPING OTHERS. It has been conclusively proven that when an individual in recovery commits to helping someone else begin and to maintain recovery, that there is much less chance of re-lapse. Be consistent in all that you do.

Congratulations. You have just mastered one of the most powerful mental and emotional techniques on planet earth!

There are many other benefits to fasting (both physically and spiritually), that you should educate yourself in. I will cover most of these benefits in my fasting manual which will soon be published.

In the next chapter we will witness the inner struggle of an individual attempting to reprogram a memory from childhood. It is a story in which I struggled with inde-cision as whether or not it should be written and shared. I decided that it should be written.

It was not an easy story to write.

It is my personal story.

Chapter Ten

The Little Boy with a Tail

As a troubled teenager in search for truth, I eventually found my answer in a Spirit filled experience with Jesus Christ. From that moment on my life dramatically changed. I am not saying that it has all been a bed of roses, but I have always known that the Rose of Sharon was with me, and that has been enough.

There were a couple of especially dark valleys I experienced in my walk, and during those valleys I seemed to revert back to a mode of handling things that seemed out of place compared to my usual modus operandi. Especially notable was the fact that during those dark trials I began to experience nightmares which repeatedly occurred each and every single night. Even long after the trial was over, although it was no longer nightly, I periodically would experience the nightmare again. The nightmare would suddenly begin by discovering I was lost. I would be in the dark, in some unknown location, somewhere in the wilderness. A huge silhouette of a towering figure was crashing through the wilderness in pursuit of me. I managed to stay one step ahead of it, but it always seemed to be closing in on me. I had committed some unknown wrong for which the towering shadow was pursuing me. In the nightmare I felt as though the world had turned against me, that I was despised and hated. Feelings of worthlessness and anxiety flooded me. As I crouched in the darkness, I knew I had to go back and "undo" something, or to make something right, before the horrible shadow caught me. If I made it right, whatever it was that needed to be made right, then all would be well again. I always woke up just as the monstrous shadow hovered over me.

I was sure that this reoccurring nightmare, which contained a detailed pattern of thinking and emotions, was rooted in some memory that was probably still slumbering somewhere in the depth of my hidden mind.

One day I decided to employ the fasting method in order to dredge up the original root of these strange valley experiences.

Several times I went to a quiet place of prayer and contemplated the origin of these feelings. An experience that I had gone through very early in life persistently came back to me. I believed this was the original root of the discomfort. That "DVD" needed deleted.

A LONG TIME AGO

My fathers early history can be described as "from rags to riches and back to rags again." After marrying my mother he became prosperous in a very short period of time. He soon owned a ranch with many acres of land, he owned his own oil wells, had several hired hands, cattle, and race horses which he both raised and raced. On the property he also had a gasoline station and a small gro-

147

cery store which he hired others to operate. He was a licensed barber and also had a barber shop on the property which was opened part time.

I was probably around three years old, when I remember my father arguing with one of the hired hands. To this day I can't recall exactly what the argument was about, but I do know that shortly after the argument he ordered the hired hand to tie up one of his prize horses. Soon afterward, the air was filled with the alarming neighing of a frightened horse as it stood high on its hind legs. Dust was swirling through the air as the horse violently struggled. I recall Mother shouting for Father to rescue the horse and he shouted back that he couldn't do anything, because he couldn't get close enough to the violently frightened animal to loosen the rope. I was to later learn that the hired hand, still upset over the argument, went to tie up the horse as he was ordered, but instead of tying it up properly by using the bridle, he instead made a noose with a slip knot, placed it around the horse's neck, and then spooked it. As the horse struggled to get away, the slip knot grew tighter and tighter and the animal eventually hung itself. I remember the horse finally falling to the ground, flailing in the dust, struggling, and finally collapsing. I remember Father setting by it and holding its head on his lap. I don't recall too much of anything else except for Mother asking him something and he replied that it was just too late. He loved this horse and it was quite evident the death devastated him. He picked up a shovel and began to dig a hole right where it had just died. I remember getting a shovel and trying to help him. I know I must have just been in the way. Someone commented that it would take all day to bury the horse and Father said he didn't care how long it took. I don't know if he finished digging the hole and burying it that same evening or the next, but I do recall the sun setting in the horizon, and with tear misted eyes he placed a home made wooden tombstone at the head of the grave with the animals name inscribed on it. He must have been so exhausted that night.

The first opportunity he had, he went to the local Sheriff and told what the hired hand had done. He was to soon learn that the Sheriff of this very small farming community was best friends with the hired hands parents. After hearing the story, the Sheriff is said to have laughed about it in my father's face. Outraged, my father left the Sheriff's office determined to see justice served. I am uncertain how soon after the confrontation with the Sheriff that he did it, but he took a truck and went to the property, on which the hired hand and his family lived, herded up a few of his cattle, and headed with them out of state. He took them to an auction in a neighboring state to sell, in an attempt to retrieve the money he had lost on his horse.

He never made it home from the auction.

My memory is hazy as to exactly what happened next, but I can still hear the horrific, frightening wail of my mother being informed of my father's incarceration. Sometime later I was sitting beside Mother in a courtroom. The judge said something, I believe it was my fathers sentencing to prison, and Mother burst forth wailing in tears. I then jumped up, stood on the seat of my chair, raised my hand and pointed my finger straight at the judge, and in defense of my parents I bravely shouted to the top of my voice, *"You are a bad, bad man!! You better leave my Mommy and Daddy alone!!!"*

149

Of course I had no idea of what was really going on. I remember going to the prison and looking through a little smudgy glass window and trying to tell Father I loved him and wanted him home. I remember to this very day the tear in his eye and the pain that swept across his weary face.

Mother knew nothing about running the ranch or any of the other businesses. I do not know the details or how it happened, but somehow everything ended up in my grandfather's name and he began to take care of the businesses. My grandfather, my mothers father, was a shrewd business man. He manipulated the situation and moved Mother and I into his home with Grandma and himself, and sold my father's ranch, his home, the oil wells, and everything he had ever owned. He convinced Mother that was the best way to handle it and he would give them back the money made on the property, with interest, when her husband returned home from prison. It was later said his true desire was to make his daughter dependent upon him, and hopefully he could eventually persuade her to divorce her husband. At any rate, when Father finally was released to return home for his family, he asked Grandpa where all of his money was. Grandpa replied that he had kept the money to take care of room and board for keeping his wife and kids while he was incarcerated. My father had lost everything he had ever owned.

I have no idea how long he was incarcerated. Mother said six months to a year. Father said over two years. Mother was embarrassed about his time spent and therefore most probably minimized it. Father, in later years, was a storyteller extraordinairé, who probably exaggerated the time spent for the sake of giving the story more

of a touch of drama. Most probably the truth is somewhere in between. Another family member recently informed me that it was a year and a half, which is probably closer to the truth. To a little boy it seemed like decades.

All I know for certain is that we went to live with
Florence, my grandmother, and Merle, my grandfather,
on their farm. While Grandma was one of the most precious women who ever walked the earth, my grandfather
was Satan incarnate. He was a lean, tall man, partially
bald with silver hair. He had piercing eyes and a commanding, irritating voice. When he became angry, fire
shot from his eyes and demons rode the winds of his
voice. He was like a mad man poised to kill. Fear would
energize the atmosphere like electricity and everything
around or near him would shrink in horror. One local le-
gend about him says he was working in the field one day
with a mule. The mule became stubborn and refused to
move. Grandpa became so outraged at the animal that
he bent down and savagely bit a large chunk out of the
mule's ear. His children all suffered with anxiety as a
result of being raised around him. At the age of three or
four years old I was sent to live with my loving grandfather. It was like living with Hannibal Lector.

I was not allowed to play and was constrained to talk in
a whisper. I had seen the pictures in a comic book, that
my mother had read to me, about a mouse that picked up
his backpack and went on a journey. That night I
dreamed I was in Heaven. Jesus and Mother were watching me and smiling. I was a little mouse in Heaven and
they were observing me, as I enjoyed myself scurrying
through the golden palace of Heaven. Jesus, for my
pleasure, had temporarily turned me into a mouse. The

next morning I wanted to pretend I was a mouse. A mouse, you see, could scurry around unnoticed, having fun without someone screaming at it. A mouse would be almost invisible. I got an empty pillow case for my back-pack, and with a safety pin and a string, I made myself a tail and began to crawl around on the floor pretending I was a mouse. Grandpa was setting in his easy chair with his newspaper, as usual, propped in front of him. In retrospect he resembled the wicked witch of the West as he sat there with his nose stuck in that newspaper. As I crawled around the floor, the space between the back of his chair and the wall seemed inviting. It looked like a dark little alley or tunnel where a mouse would wish to crawl through. My little hands and knees carried me scurrying across the floor with my little string tail behind me. As I went behind his chair I was startled by the piercing roar of Grandpa's voice as he threateningly screamed at me for going behind his chair. Mother anxiously ran into the room. Grandpa leaped to his feet in blazing anger, the newspaper rustling like leaves in a tornado as he vented heated rage at my blatant tres-passing of his kingdom! I suddenly felt terror. I realized I wasn't supposed to go behind his chair. I had done a bad thing. I had entered and crawled through this space be-hind his chair. To my infantile mind the only obvious thing to do was to turn around and go back the way that I had come and "undo" what I had done. He didn't like me coming from the right of his chair and emerging on the left of it? I'll just turn around and go back to the right side where I entered and reverse my journey. That should make him happy. Right? Because I went behind the chair again, he screamed even louder. Hiroshima paled beside his furious explosion. I do not remember all of his words exactly but I knew for certain he was going to kill me. I remember hearing Mothers strained fearful voice, *"Oh, Curt, why did you go back around his chair? Why?"* Grandma was trying to calm Grandpa telling him he would have a heart attack if he didn't *"settle himself."* Shaking and trembling I leaped to my feet. Grandpa was screaming obscenities at me and going for a switch with which to beat me.

I ran.

I had no idea where I was going but I ran.

And I ran, and I ran, and I ran.

Mother couldn't have rescued me anymore than Grandpa could have caught me. The world blurred before my eyes.

Grandpa's large old country home was nestled at the edged of the woodland. Dashing into the woods I eventually came to a steep, rocky hill. I climbed over the rocks and stones until I found a rock I could crouch down behind and feel safe. I was far enough away that wherever I was, I could no longer hear his emotionally assaulting threats. Crumpled up tight against the rock, I wept. After I finally quit trembling I just sat. I sat immobile for hours and hours. I sat there all day. The sun began to set and darkness fell. I feared what creatures might be lurking in that darkness but no matter how horrific such creatures may prove to be, none was more terrifying then Grandpa. I was bad. I was no good. Grandpa was tired of having this bad, no good little boy around and he was going to kill him. He was going to mercilessly beat him. He was going to scream with his face blood red and his eyes protruding from their sockets and devour me with his terrifying wrath.

The heat of the day exchanged its day shift duties over to the cool and gentle, almost undetectable, breezes of the night. The sounds of the woodland creatures began to serenade the gradual changing of the guard. I don't remember, but I am sure that in the unified concert of crickets and whip-poor-wills was the call of a lonely hoot owl or two. I sat there a long time in the darkness, clutching the rock, as the hours slowly passed by. It seemed like forever.

I decided to emerge from the rock I was hiding behind and head toward the edge of the hill.

Then through the darkness of the fearful night I heard the angelic voice of my mother calling my name.

There are no words to describe what I felt in that moment.

I stumbled over rocks I could no longer see and made my way toward the voice. I ran through the woods with branches slapping my face and vines reaching out to entangle my little feet, but I continued to run toward the voice of safety.

Then I saw a light shine in the darkness.

I ran toward the light.

I rushed into Mothers arms so fast I probably almost tumbled her. Her arms of love and security let me know I had survived.

I had survived, Grandpa, I had survived the rocky cliffs, I had survived the woods, I had survived the unknown creatures of night, but most of all I had survived my own paralyzing fear. I was safe again.

But Grandpa was still watching me. A day would come when . . .

There would be a time when he would . . .

Well, I didn't know just exactly what he would do — but I knew it would be terrifying. It seemed to involve something about the end of the world.

Mother had tried to rescue me when Grandpa began to chase me. It had just happened so quickly. I had escaped so fast. Also Mother was just as petrified with fear in Grandpas presence as was everyone else. She had no where to go, no where to take her family, and the traumatic memories Grandpa had implanted in her were playing and telling her Grandpa was in control.

I was never really sure what happened to me in that moment of my life. I was to later experience more terrifying experiences but somehow this one, being my first brush with terror, became a root of fear that eventually other crawling vines grew out of.

EXPLORING THE TRAUMA

After identifying the trauma, it seemed almost impossible to take even the first of the nine steps. A young man had come to my home pleading for help. He was hopelessly hooked on drugs and needed detoxed. Unable to get him into any of the local detox units, he was determined to become clean and went through detox in my home. The withdrawals were horrendous.

155

At the same time I was preparing for a trip to the Middle East. I was going into the Palestinian West Bank. I was also preparing to take biblical literature into Syria and Iraq. There were missionary works in Israel where I was not only ministering, but was hoping to gather important information for a book I am writing on the history of the Church. In addition to all of that were my ordinary daily duties, my duties in the local church, and my duties as both a father and a husband. Believe me; if anyone had excuses not to create a treatment plan, set a date for the sessions, and to prepare a safe place for the sessions, I had it. I made up my mind not to be deterred.

I began to prepare for my fast. On the second day of my fast I identified the traumatic memory concerning my grandfather. I identified the negative belief and the negative statement programming. In my safe place I locked the door and decided to sit on the floor with my back against the door. This made me feel even safer.

Then suddenly, I experienced a twinge of fear. Grandpa was not someone I wanted to visit.

A TRIP TO GRANDPA'S HOUSE

I closed my eyes. I prayed. I listened.

I asked for protection upon me as I journeyed inward. I felt a great peace.

I went to the beginning of the trauma. I lingered there until I could "see" the scenery, "feel" the feelings, and re-experience the "thoughts" of the original experience. It was there. No doubt about it, it was there. Like a DVD in high definition, the scene began to play. At the beginning of the scene with Grandpa, I recalled sitting by the hallway door on the floor playing with my stuffed toys. I had never remembered that before. I could smell a faint musty scent in the old farm house. It must have been early because I could now see the sun rising from the east window, casting its golden brilliance across the hardwood floor. I had a string pinned to the back of my little pair of jeans pretending it was a tail. Grandpa seemed engrossed in his newspaper and would surely not notice a little mouse crawl behind his chair. As I crawl behind his chair I hear Grandpa's terrible scream . . . then something happened . . . the "DVD" froze. There was no more scream, no more crawling . . . just a scene frozen in time. I reversed the memory slightly and proceeded again. Grandpa had kicked back the chair before he screamed. I never recalled that before. When he kicked back the chair it prevented me from exiting the other side. He continued screaming for me to get out. I informed him that I couldn't and that his chair was blocking me. He screamed, *"Then go back the same way you went!"*

There was the key.

I had never remembered him making that statement before.

He moved his chair up, and I exited the direction I had been going, but then TURNED AROUND to *"go back the way I went!"* He screamed even more thinking I was just rebelling against his orders.

I had gone through a dark place trailing a long tail behind me. It turned out I was doing a "bad" thing. Grandpa Meryl suggested I *"go back the way I went"* which my infantile mind defined as reversing the wrong direction by retracing my steps and doing it over. There was a certain way Grandpa wanted it done. I was confused as to exactly what that way was because when I did it he screamed even more. I ran. I gave it all I had within me. Even as I relived the event I could still feel the branches slapping my face, the rocks under my bare feet, and my heart beating just as fast and as hard as it could. I ran and ran and hid in the woods until darkness fell. I relived the loneliness, the fear, and the insecurity. I found myself thinking the very same thoughts in the very same way I had created them as a child of three or four years old. Only now I was observing those thoughts through more mature lenses. I began to understand things in a way I had never understood before. Mother had been frantically searching for me and had at last wandered into the area I had fled to. Mother finally coming to my rescue was the only positive imprint in the memory. It is because of the root of that one positive memory, in the midst of a negative experience, that I developed an unmovable determination that no matter how dark the wilderness, or how impossible the situation seems, I WILL make it.

A NIGHTMARE ON MERLE'S STREET

My reoccurring nightmares suddenly made sense. The nightmare would suddenly begin by my discovering I was lost in the dark in some unknown location somewhere in the wilderness. My inner child was still experiencing being lost in the woods because it had LITERALLY been lost in the woods beyond Grandpa's farm. The huge silhouette of a towering figure that was crashing through the wilderness in pursuit of me was the towering figure of my grandfather. The unknown wrong,

158

for which the towering shadow was pursuing me, was the act of crawling behind his chair. In the nightmare I felt as though the world had turned against me, that I was despised and that I was hated because I had accepted Grandpa's words and actions that had portrayed this belief to me. This belief resulted in the feelings of low self esteem, depression, and anxiety that flooded me in the dream. In the nightmare I crouched in the darkness, knowing I had to go back and "undo" something that I had done wrong. I never knew exactly what it was that needed to be made right, but if I could "redo" it the right way, then all would be well again . . . I would finally be "perfect." I now realized I was feeling the childhood concept Grandpa had inadvertently instilled in me, *"Go back the same way you went!"*

Of course . . . if the child could go back the same way he went, perhaps he could get it just "right" the next time around.

The above experience was a basic root of a weed-like vine in my garden. Later in life other traumatic experiences occurred and other weeds began to grow. These new weeds became a support the original vine could grow and wrap around. Other vines and weeds grew, each dependent upon the other for support, all going back to the original vine.

GRANDPA, WHAT BIG TEETH YOU HAVE

I had always said I loved my grandfather and never spoke of him with anything but reverence. It was sort of like a Holocaust survivor saying, *"I love Hitler."* It didn't make sense. One day I was chatting with a friend of mine, which happened to be a clinical psychologist, and I mentioned my grandfather's antics but ended saying, *"but I loved my grandfather."* My friend looked at me and replied, *"Why? He sounds like an #*#*#*# to me!"*

Something happened to me that moment. I suddenly realized that I did NOT love my grandfather. I was living a lie. Inwardly I despised the man. However, this was not an acceptable emotion to have toward my mother's father. Therefore the energy of the hatred was reversed into a pseudo-feeling of love. It was a classic reaction formation.

Of course my religious training had taught me one must not hate.

It also taught me one must not lie.

And denying my negative feelings toward Grandpa was indeed a big, black, festering lie!

UNMASKING THE BIG BAD . . . "TIGER"

I went to the beginning of the memory again. I wept. I poured out every expression of fear the event produced. I expressed every emotion involved. Then I went back again. This time I faced Grandfather. I screamed at him, *"I despise you! I don't want to, but I do! I feel anger toward you for scaring a little boy to death, for making my life miserable, for making me think I was worthless, and for making me nervous and anxious!"* Of course I knew it was my reaction and NOT Grandfather which had produced these feelings, but at this point I was simply expressing the raw emotions my inner child had felt from that experience.

I went back to the beginning of the memory and this time as I went through it I screamed my positive belief programming into it. *"I am NOT worthless! I do NOT have to be perfect! I am a child of the King and that is enough!"* I reprogrammed my positive statement into it. *"I am not perfect but GREATER IS HE THAT IS IN ME THEN HE THAT IS IN THE WORLD!"* I shouted it over and over gain until I felt that the scripture had penetrated my mind and soul.

Afterward I forgave Grandpa.

After decades of pain from a man who had in reality been lying six feet under the ground most of those years, I finally forgave him.

Words cannot explain the change that took place when I let it go.

It seemed as though a cumbrous load, that had been fastened to me for decades, had finally been lifted. It was as if heavy, metal chains had suddenly turned to dust and crumbled. I felt free. I felt released. I felt clean and new. I forgave him.

I was reminded of the song by Brandon Heath, "I'm Not Who I Was":

> *I wish you could see me now,*
> *I wish I could show you how,*
> *I'm not who I was.*
> *I used to be mad at you.*
> *A little on the hurt-side too,*
> *But I'm not who I was.*

I found my way around,
to forgiven' you,

some-time-ago,
But I never got to tell you . . .

I found us in a photograph,
I saw me and I had to laugh,
Ya' know, I'm not who I was.
Oh there you were right above me,
and I wonder if you ever loved me.
Just for who I was.

When the pain came back again;
like a bitter friend.
It was all that I could do,
To keep myself from blaming you . . .

. . . But the thing that I find most amazing,
in amazing grace,
Is the chance to give it out,
Maybe that's what love is all about.
I wish you could see me now,
I wish I could show you how,
I'm not who I was. [47]

After my session I went downstairs, put on some soft classical music, and totally exhausted I fell into a very deep sleep.

I found myself lost in the dark.

I was in the woods.

162

A towering dark shadow came crashing through the foliage toward me.

For the first time in decades of experiencing this dream I did not run. I had no reason to run. I was no longer afraid.

The dark menacing shadow stood over me. I quietly stood up, and I spoke to it, *"I'm not afraid anymore, Grandpa. I forgave you."*

The shadow then quietly backed away and disappeared forever into the night.

To this very day I have never had that nightmare again.

I can confidently say it will never return.

After many decades Grandpa now rests in peace . . . and I, after many decades, have turned everything over to the Prince of Peace.

Chapter Eleven

It Works if You Work It

SHAUN

Shaun had spent his entire life in the state of depression.

I had met Shaun years ago while working with John Bradshaw. Although John had authored several best sellers, including "The Homecoming," and had thousands of admirers, he was one of the most humble men I have ever had the privilege of knowing. No one he met was less or more important than anyone else. I truly believe he had a genuine compassion for others. John Bradshaw's work was not of an exclusively Christian nature, but he repeatedly expressed to me his love for the Lord. His workshops consisted of group counseling sessions in which one would do "inner child" work. I was assisting John in some workshops in Cincinnati and was facilitating the inner child sessions when one man began to collapse with grief. I took him aside and John, who ordinarily was unable to spend a inordinate length of time with just one individual, devoted a great amount of time to

164

this one man. Afterward, back in the dressing room, I went to see how John was doing. His eyes were filled with compassion. He told me that the man we had worked with was one of the most *"messed up"* people he had ever encountered.

Shaun was in so much pain that I am not certain he could even fully concentrate or effectively be a part of the workshops. John and I did all we could for him but evidently it wasn't destiny for him to face his hidden horrors at this time.

Before leaving Cincinnati I got the mans telephone number and address. I had communicated with him afterward but never really received a response.

Years passed by and one day I remembered Shaun. I went through some old files my wife had wished many times I would have disposed of and there, amongst volumes of useless information, was Shaun's telephone number and address. When I called the number I was told it was not Shaun's number but it now belonged to a relative of Shaun. The chances of the number leading me to Shaun after several years had passed seemed very slim, so I took this almost as a sign that I was indeed supposed to contact him. Shaun's number was not available to me but I was provided with an email address. I emailed him and waited for several days.

YOU'VE GOT MAIL

I thought Shaun had either not received the message, didn't remember me, or just didn't want to respond. Then one day I checked my mail and he had answered me.

165

Nothing had really changed. He was still in a perpetual depression and had remained there for all of these years. He remembered John Bradshaw and he thought he remembered who I was. I shared with him what fasting could accomplish and how the method worked.

Time passed by and again I thought he had dismissed my email. Then I got another email from him requesting more information. I mailed him all the material and instructions I had. Nothing is without some element of risk with someone someplace in the world — not even the fasting method. To protect myself I encouraged him to seek his physician and therapist before proceeding with the method. Again there was a space of silence.

One day Shaun contacted me. He was completely overjoyed. He said he had tried every therapy and medication known to man and never one time experienced relief. He informed me he had followed the instructions to the "T" and that during his fasting session that a raging river of pain flowed from his innermost being. He said for the first time in his life he actually revisited the painful past as though he were there, addressed his abusers as though they were there, and was now living his life as though they never were!

The last time Shaun contacted me he was still free from depression. He said there were several memories, each connected with the other, that had also been discharged but he had now put them all behind him. He was at last, after decades —actually for the first time in his entire life— waking up in the morning without the dark cloud of depression hanging over him.

Shaun says he is now free from his past.

TONY

Tony was no stranger to depression and anxiety. He too had suffered from perfectionism. He was tormented day and night by thoughts that he may have sinned. He would remember something he did decades ago and, not remembering if he had thoroughly repented and cleansed himself of that particular sin, he would go into a panic and begin to ceremonially purge himself. If he drove by a billboard portraying a seductive woman or advertising an alcoholic beverage, he would feel the need to cleanse himself either with an anointing oil or, in a severe case, to be re-baptized. Sometimes Tony was so overwhelmed by his constant moment to moment need for total spiritual purity that he would collapse under pressure and intentionally go "look" at the billboards that were "contaminating" him or to think the thoughts that made him "impure" just so he would "know" for sure that he had "sinned" which made it easier to "know" he was actually "*repenting* of sin" when he repented, was anointed with oil, or re-baptized. Sometimes his struggle with the passion to obtain holiness became so bizarre that he lost complete contact with what was real in the world and what was not real.

When Tony discovered the fasting method he immediately began to go through the sessions. The last time I heard from Tony he was free for the first time in his life from the obsessive and compulsive behavior that had dominated, and almost destroyed, much of his life.

"I have tried EVERYTHING," Tony said. *"For the first time in my life I have found relief. I have found the answer. I have never been the same since that last fast. It is almost like being reborn. I feel new again."*

167

WILL

Will was quite a character. Suffering from intense anxiety and a dark, foreboding, low self image, Will continually made a mess of his life. He couldn't speak a single sentence without stuttering and bungling all the words up and creating comical statements that caused people to roar at him in laughter. This only served to make Will even more anxious.

His inability to talk to others led to isolation, humiliation, drugs, alcohol, pornography, and eventually to feelings of suicide.

Will was raised in the foothills of the Appalachia Mountains in a specific area where therapy and psychologists were considered *"of the devil"* or at the very least *"nonsense."* Using the fasting method in a clinical setting would have set up red flags for Will.

However the beautiful thing about the fasting method is that it DOES NOT REQUIRE A CLINICAL SETTING!

It CAN be used in a clinical and a therapeutic setting but it is not necessary. It has only been outlined in a scientific way in this book, in order that the reader may understand the specifics in an organized, systematical way.

The method has been used for THOUSANDS OF YEARS outside of a clinical setting. Moses, Elijah, Daniel, Christ, Paul . . . none of these fasted in a counselors office!!!

Will finally came to the Lord but even after he was filled with the Spirit he continued suffering from low self esteem, troublesome memories from the past, and incoherent stuttering. He was instructed to seek his deliverance and healing by doing the following:

1. Set aside a time and place for prayer.
2. Begin the fast.
3. Identify the memory and the negative belief that the enemy planted in your mind. Identify a positive belief and a scripture to replace it with.
4. Begin praying a fervent prayer before the Lord.
5. Explore the troublesome memory and the negative self image, or damaging belief, involved in the memory. Be honest and open before God.
6. Let go of the guilt and pain of the past. Cry out to God! Tell him exactly how you feel! Rebuke the poisonous seed the enemy planted in that memory.
7. Replace the memory and the belief with the new understanding of it that the Spirit has revealed to you. Firmly quote the scripture you previously chose. Fervently acknowledge your new understanding of the memory to God! Acknowledge fervently to him how determined and sincere you are about this! Allow forgiveness and healing to take place.
8. Terminate the fast gradually with proper foods.
9. Create a schedule for Bible reading, prayer, church attendance, and other lifestyle changes.

HMMM . . . do these nine steps sound familiar?

They should.

They are the very exact same nine steps lined out earlier in this book — but without the technical details.

And IT WORKED!!!

The young man that once could not speak a sentence without stuttering, the young man whose speech got so turned around that he was ridiculed by his friends, the same person who was afraid to speak to people . . . that same man is now IN THE MINISTRY!!!

The young man who once had difficulty speaking a single sentence just one on one now speaks before great crowds!

He calls the FIAR fasting method the "FIRE fasting method" because for him it stirred up the Holy Ghost fire which burned out the dross of the past!

What a change! What a miracle! The Bible has proven not to be outdated as many would have us believe!

Fasting was relevant then, and it is still relevant in the twenty first century!

For thousands of years many have utilized the scriptural practice of fasting and prayer with remarkable results. While acknowledging the spiritual benefits of fasting, we must ask ourselves if the psychotherapeutic effects have been present in fasting as well? The sages taught that man consists of a body, a mind (soul), and a spirit — it now appears evident that fasting attends to the healing of all three! No wonder so many have found deliverance in fasting and prayer! FIAR fasting is effective but it is

170

miraculously effective when empowered by prayer!

This wonderful gift of fasting not only provided healing for mans body, mind and spirit in biblical days but is readily accessible to you today. It worked for Will — and what it has done for others, it can do for you.

ROBERT

Robert, whom we met in chapter two, was so devastated by the memory of his father beating his mother that he experienced chronic depression from that time forward. Robert heard his father threaten to kill his mother and then witnessed her beaten to unconsciousness as she was covered with her own blood. After his father found him the next morning and brought him downstairs, he remembers the whole family sitting around the table, smiling like hypocrites, and pretending they were one whole happy family. It took a few days for the bruises on his mothers face to heal but the bruises on Roberts heart were to never heal from that experience.

If you recall, we previously related how Robert had a part of his skull removed,using a drill from the hardware store, in attempt to find relief from debilitating depression. Sadly the hole was not large enough for the huge amount of pain to escape through. The answer was not to drill a hole in his head but to heal a hole in his heart.

Robert was located and briefed about the nature of trauma and the possibility of the fasting method as an answer to assisting in alleviating the pain of his personal trauma. Robert expressed an interest in the method. An extensive manuscript detailing the method was sent to him with the encouragement to share it with his health care provider.

Robert fasted employing the method described. He was ecstatic with the initial results. However a few days later the depression returned. He used the fasting method a second time. This time there was very little if any results at all. Determined to end his lifelong battle with depression he went on two successive fasts with a one day interval in between and his final results were nothing less than remarkable.

Robert, for the first time in his entire life, was free from chronic depression.

Friends tried to discourage him by maintaining his relief was only temporary and the depression would come back.

Days went by, weeks went by, month's passed, and Father Time slowly kept walking on. During the entire time friends kept insisting the chronic depression would return.

It never did.

Robert tells the world he is cured. The doctors tell him there is no such thing as a cure for depression.

Robert doesn't care WHAT they think . . . for the first time in his life he is enjoying his life.

As far as Robert is concerned . . . that's a cure.

Chapter Twelve

The Voice of Hope

My heart hurts for the untold number of people needlessly suffering from the pain of the past.

I know this method works and it is my desire to share it with others that they too may find relief.

Many times I have pondered on the existence of pain in the world. Why was it even created?

The world-famous leprosy surgeon, Dr. Paul Brand, spent most of his life caring for the forsaken lepers in India. His greatest discovery was learning that those with leprosy didn't lose their extremities due to the flesh simply falling off. He discovered that what they lacked was the ability to feel physical sensations. Restricted blood flow to the extremities caused the nerve endings to die. They could no longer sense pain. As a result they lost fingers and toes to fire, sharp objects, and other daily accidents.

The greatest mystery of all was how the lepers could go

to sleep and then wake up the next morning with missing fingers and toes that could never be found. These appendages had not fallen to the floor nor could they be found in the lepers bedding.

Dr. Brand was determined to solve the mystery. He stationed people to watch them as they slept and, to their surprise, they discovered that rats were coming in and nibbling off their fingers and toes. Feeling no pain, they never woke up to brush the rats away. For their well being the good doctor made it mandatory that they took cats with them wherever they slept.

He also discovered they went blind simply because they could not feel the discomfort that caused most people to blink their eyes.

The doctor observed foot injuries in which an ankle turned, tearing muscles and tendons, but the leper would simply adjust and walk with a crooked gait. There was no pain warning the individual to rest the ankle or to seek any sort of treatment for it.

Well known athletes have permanently damaged their bodies by numbing their throbbing, debilitating injuries with painkillers and injections and then running out on the field while still injured.

Ironically we should be thankful for pain. In the long run it allows us to avoid further damage to ourselves.

However many ignore their hurt or desperately try to numb it.

Even as you read these words, countless numbers of people are trying to numb their despair with drugs and alcohol. Their families are suffering. Many are fleeing ghosts from the past and the hurt inside that prevents them from achieving the good things in life they could achieve. Millions are trying to escape the very hurt that is trying to alert them that something is wrong in their lives.

When you injure or burn yourself, pain is natural. When my wife Rebecca was a child she placed her hand on the side of a pot bellied stove. In shock she immediately withdrew her blistered hand. The pain served a purpose. The pain was a message. The message was, *"You are touching something that is harming you. Remove your hand from it and do not touch it again in the future!"* Without this message she would possibly have left her hand there until it was no longer usable.

Pain serves a purpose. Pain is a "message." The message is saying, *"Something is wrong. Do something about it."*

If you are experiencing pain, depression, or remorse, you can rest assure that the message it is sending you serves a purpose. It is telling you that something is wrong. It is telling you to do something about it before it is too late.

Continual pain is not natural.

Continual hurt and despair is the result of unsolved inner conflicts, fears, damaged emotions, or trauma from the past. It is present to alert you to the fact that the inner conflicts that you have never effectively addressed are still there inflicting their damage upon your life, adversely influencing major decisions and choices you make, and shaping the way you view and interact with the world around you. Do not ignore the message. Do not wait until the root of your hurt and dysfunction consumes your whole life and destroys those closest to you.

Find someone to confide in.

Make an appointment with your clergy or with a counselor or, even better, with both. Most importantly find a place of prayer and speak to the *"Wonderful Counselor"* (Isa.9:6).

Whatever you do, you must NOT ignore pain. It is a message that something is wrong and it is there to remind you to do something about it.

Talk to your counselor, clergy, or physician about the fasting method. It may be the very lifeline you are seeking for. Many have discovered, with great joy, this precious technique that has stood the test of time and provided deliverance when all other methods have failed.

In the wise book wherein we discovered the fasting phenomenon — that ancient manuscript we call the Holy Bible — is another gem of wisdom inscribed by the Apostle Paul, who wrote, *"This one thing I do, forgetting those things which are behind."* (Phil 3:13).

The problem is that most people have not put their problems *"behind"* them. They carry them with them every day of their life. The undeleted DVD of the traumatic experience is preserved and protected within them. I implore you to dig that memory out, discharge and reprogram the space it once occupied and then forever PUT IT BEHIND YOU!

Don't look back. Let it go. Live life to the fullest.

Science has long labored in search for an answer.

The answer has not been found in a test tube.

The answer has not been found in a research study.

The answer has not been found in trepanation, lobotomy, electric shock treatments, excessive medication, rapid eye movements, mesmerism, hypnotism, psychoanalysis, or a host of other therapeutic theories.

The answer is contained within the pages of that ancient manuscript written many, many years ago.

Times have changed.

Methods have changed.

Men have changed.

The manuscript and its message have never changed.

It is time we pause and listen to its ancient voice.

Finis

References

[1] IMS Health, National Prescription Audit Plus, National Disease and Therapeutic Index, years 1998 to 2002, Data extracted 1/ 2004

[2] World Health Organization

[3] Http;//www.drugtext.org/library/books/recreationaldrugs/tranquilizers.htm

[4] Westfield, John Cloud, Time Magazine, 2/26/2001

[5] Boodman, Sandra G., The Washington Post, 9/24/96, pg Z14.

[6] Lyons, Tom, Canadian Press, Sat., 9/28/2002

[7] The Washington Post, April 6, 1980, Sunday, Final Edition
SECTION: First Section; A1, HEADLINE: Psychosurgery's Effects Still Linger;Benefits of Psychosurgery Still Debated by Doctors; After 20 Years, Effects of the Lobotomy Era Still Linger

[8] Cott MD, Alan, Contribution, The Center for the Improvement of Human Functioning Intl. (CIHFI0 2004)

[9] Cott, Allan, Jerome Agel, Eugene Boe, Fasting; the ultimate Diet, 1981, ISBN 9780553200652

[10] Shapiro, Francine, PHD, Eye Movement Desensitation and Reprocessing: Basic Principles, Protocols and Procedures, Guilford Press, New York, 2001 (2nd ed.)

[11] Michell, John, Eccentric Lives & Peculiar Notions, Black Dog & Leventhal Publishers, (2/11/2002)

[12] Shimelpfening, Nancy, Trepanation, About.com, 8/25/2008, reviewed by Dr. Steven Gans, MD

[13] International Trepanation Advocacy Group (ITAG), Inc. P. O. Box 65, Wernersville, PA 19565

[14] Shelton, Herbert, The Fine Art and Science of Fasting, Natural Hygiene Press, 1978. Dr. Gina Shaw, MA, Fasting for Health, article, 10/18/08.

[15] Encyclopædia Britannica. 2008. Encyclopædia Britannica Online. 07 Oct. 2008

[16] McManamy, John, The Father of Lobotomy, 2/12/2008

[17] Kessler, Ronald. The Sins of the Father: Joseph P. Kennedy and the Dynasty He Founded. New York: Warner Books, 1997, p. 246

179

[18] Kessler, p. 237

[19] Kessler, p. 224

[20] Kessler, p. 227

[21] Kessler, p. 232–235

[22] Kessler, p. 232–235

[23] Sutherland J. (2004) Should they de-Nobel Moniz? The Guardian. London

[24] Mark Durand & David H. Barlow (2006),Essentials of Abnormal Psychology, 4th ed.", Thomson Wadsworth.

[25] Tooth GC, and Newton, MP: Leukotomy in England and Wales 1942-1954. London, Her Majesty's Stationary Office, 1961

[26] Baer, L., et al. (1995). Cingulotomy for intractable obsessive-compulsive disorder. Archives of General Psychiatry, 52, 384-392

[27] Kaplan and Sadock (1997)

[28] Smith, Andrew, Newsday coverage of Paul Henri Thomas, March 3, 2001, His New Battle, Patient takes fight against electric shock treatment to court

[29] MacQueen, Geoff , Miner and News, April 28, 2001

[30] Out of Mind Magazine, October 1998

[31] Burgher, Valerie, Newsday, July 22, 2001

[32] Mosher, Jim , Kenora Enterprise, July 20, 1997

[33] Burgher, Valerie, Newsday, July 22, 2001

[34] Burgher, Valerie, Newsday, July 22, 2001

[35] HELSLEY, SCOTT, PH.D., TASMINA SHEIKH, M.D., KYE Y. KIM, M.D., and S.K. PARK, M.D.,Buffalo, N.Y. The American Journal of Psychiatry, 1999

[36] Sutherland SM, Davidson Jr., Department of Psychiatry, Duke University Medical Center, Durham, North Carolina)

[37] Solomon SD, Gerrity ET, Muff AM: Efficacy of treatments for posttraumatic stress disorder. JAMA 1992; 268:633–638

[38] S. D. Solomon, E. T. Gerrity and A. M. Muff
Division of Applied and Services Research, National Institute of Mental Health, Rockville, Md. 20857.

[39] MindFreedom International - 454 Willamette, Suite 216 - PO Box 11284 - Eugene, OR 97440-3484 USA

[40] Mattson, M. P. et al. Intermittent fasting dissociates beneficial effects of dietary restriction on glucose metabolism and neuronal resistance to injury from calorie intake. Proceedings of the National Academy of Sciences 100, 6216-6220 (May 13, 2003), Mark P. Mattson, Ph.D., Senior Investigator, Chief, Laboratory of Neurosciences and Chief, Cellular and Molecular Neurosciences Section, Article : Cheryl Simon Silver Genome News 7/9/04, Davis, Jeanie Lerche, WebMD Health News, 4/28/2004,

[41] Sato, Rebecca, The Daily Galaxy, Reboot Your Brain -The Scientific Secrets of Brain Regeneration, 10/31/2007, Anson, R. M., Guo, Z, de Cabo, R., Iyun, T., Rios, M., Hagepanos, A., Ingram, D. K., Lane, M. A. & Mattson, M. P. (2003, April 30). Intermittent fasting dissociates beneficial effects of dietary restriction on glucose metabolism and neuronal resistance to injury from calorie intake. National Academy of Sciences Online Early Edition.

[42] Marziali, Carl, USC College News of letters,arts, and sciences, March, 2008, print June 12, 2008, doi: 10.1073/pnas.0804252105 PNAS June 17, 2008 vol. 105 no. 24 8178, J. S. Valentine and E. B. Gralla, Reactive Oxygen Species Special Feature: Introduction: Reactive Oxygen Species Special Feature, Proc. Natl. Acad. Sci. USA 2008 105:8178

[43] Dodd, Gareth, Sci and Tech, China View, Study: Hungry Mice are Happy Mice, 2008-07-15 17:10:2

[44] Fontan-Lozano et al., 2007, The Journal of Neuroscience, September 19, 2007, 27(38):10185-10195; doi:10.1523/JNEUROSCI.2757-07.2007, Caloric Restriction Increases Learning Consolidation and Facilitates Synaptic Plasticity through Mechanisms Dependent on NR2B Subunits of the NMDA Receptor, Ángela Fontán-Lozano, José Luis Sáez-Cassanelli, Mari Carmen Inda, Mercedes de los Santos-Arteaga, Sergio Antonio Sierra-Domínguez, Guillermo López-Lluch, José María Delgado-García, and Ángel Manuel Carrión, División de Neurociencias y Área de Biología Celular, Universidad Pablo de Olavide de Sevilla, 41013 Sevilla, Spain

[45] Schwartz, Jeffrey M., Brain Lock: Free Yourself from Obsessive-Compulsive Behavior, Harper Perennial; 1st edition, January 31, 1997
[good trauma 134] Richard Tedeschi and Lawrence Calhoun, Post-traumatic Growth, 1996, University of North Carolina in Charlotte.

[46] Richard G. Tedeschi, Ph.D., and Lawrence Calhoun, Ph.D., "posttraumatic Growth; A New Perspective on Psychotraumatology," Psychiatric Times, April 2004

[47] Heath, Brandon, "I'm Not Who I Was," from the album "Don't Get Comfortable", Audio CD (September 19, 2006),Original Release Date: September 5, 2006 , Number of Discs: 1, Label: Reunion , ASIN: B000HEWGG0

The Fasting Phenomenon, Ward, Copyright October 2008, Revision 20, ISBN 978-0-615-26399 1

Atria Book Publishing USA AtriaBookPublishing@gmail.com

www.ingramcontent.com/pod-product-compliance
Lightning Source LLC
La Vergne TN
LVHW011349080426
835511LV00005B/209